Transnational Families

Contemporary Western society is changing and, controversially, migration is often flagged as one of the reasons. The nature of population change challenges conventional understandings of family forms and networks whilst multiculturalism poses challenges to our understanding of social change, families and social capital.

This innovative book provides an overview of the emergence of new understandings of ethnicities, identities and family forms across a number of ethnic groups, family types and national boundaries. Based on new empirical data from fairly distinct sets of transnational family networks in minority communities with a substantial presence in the United Kingdom – principally, Caribbean and Italian, but also drawing on others such as Indian – it examines their experiences and uses the concept of social capital to explore how these families manage to maintain close and meaningful links.

Transnational Families discusses, explains and illustrates the substantial problems and issues confronted by communities and families, academics and policymakers/implementers, and non-governmental organizations within a transnational world. It will be of interest to students and scholars of migration, transnationalism, families and globalization.

Harry Goulbourne is Professor of Sociology at London South Bank University, UK.

Tracey Reynolds is Senior Research Fellow in the Families & Social Capital Research Group at London South Bank University, UK.

John Solomos is Professor of Sociology at London City University, UK.

Elisabetta Zontini is Lecturer in Sociology at Nottingham University, UK.

Relationships and Resources
Series Editors: Janet Holland and Rosalind Edwards
London South Bank University

A key contemporary political and intellectual issue is the link between the relationships that people have and the resources to which they have access. When people share a sense of identity, hold similar values, trust each other and reciprocally do things for each other, this has an impact on the social, political and economic cohesion of the society in which they live. So, are changes in contemporary society leading to deterioration in the link between relationships and resources, or new and innovative forms of linking, or merely the reproduction of enduring inequalities? Consideration of relationships and resources raises key theoretical and empirical issues around change and continuity over time as well as time use, the consequences of globalization and individualization for intimate and broader social relations, and location and space in terms of communities and neighbourhoods. The books in this series are concerned with elaborating these issues and will form a body of work that will contribute to academic and political debate. Available titles include:

Marginalised Mothers
Exploring working class experiences of parenting
Val Gillies

Moving On
Bren Neale and Jennifer Flowerdew

Sibling Identity and Relationships
Sisters and brothers
Rosalind Edwards, Lucy Hadfield, Helen Laucey and Melanie Mauthner

Teenagers' Citizenship
Experiences and education
Susie Weller

Transnational Families
Ethnicities, identities and social capital
Harry Goulbourne, Tracey Reynolds, John Solomos and Elisabetta Zontini

Transnational Families
Ethnicities, identities and social capital

**Harry Goulbourne, Tracey Reynolds,
John Solomos and Elisabetta Zontini**

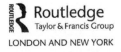
Routledge
Taylor & Francis Group

LONDON AND NEW YORK

First published 2010
by Routledge
2 Park Square, Milton Park, Abingdon, Oxfordshire OX14 4RN
Simultaneously published in the USA and Canada
by Routledge
711 Third Avenue, New York, NY 10017
Routledge is an imprint of the Taylor & Francis Group, an informa business
First issued in paperback 2011

© 2010 Harry Goulbourne, Tracey Reynolds, John Solomos and Elisabetta Zontini

Typeset in Times New Roman by
Pindar NZ, Auckland, New Zealand

British Library Cataloguing in Publication Data
A catalogue record for this book is available from the British Library

Library of Congress Cataloging-in-Publication Data
Transnational families : ethnicities, identities, and social capital / Harry
Goulbourne ... [et al.].
    p. ; cm.
  Includes bibliographical references and index.
  1. Immigrant families—Great Britain. 2. Transnationalism. 3. Families—
Cross-cultural studies. I. Goulbourne, Harry.
  [DNLM: 1. Emigrants and Immigrants. 2. Family. 3. Cross-Cultural
Comparison. 4. Ethnic Groups. HQ 519 T772 2010]
  HQ519.T727 2010
  306.85086'9120941—dc22   2009025996

ISBN 13: 978-0-415-46890-9 (hbk)
ISBN 13: 978-0-203-86218-6 (ebk)
ISBN 13: 978-0-415-67753-0 (pbk)

Contents

Acknowledgements   vi
Preface   vii

PART I
Some general questions   1

1 Theorizing transnational families   3

2 Social capital joins the trinity: families, ethnicities, communities   16

3 Methodological issues and challenges   36

4 The politics of migration   49

PART II
Living and coping across boundaries   63

5 Migrants, offspring and settlement   65

6 Families, needs and caring practices   81

7 Continuity and invention of identities within families and communities   99

8 Problems of belonging and 'return'   120

9 Alienation and escape from the family and community   136

10 Crossing boundaries: problems and opportunities in 'mixed' families   155

11 Conclusion: transnational families, policy and research challenges   177

Bibliography   182
Index   198

Acknowledgements

We have individually and collectively amassed a bundle of debt during the process of designing, researching and writing this book. We therefore take this opportunity to thank colleagues, who are too numerous to mention here, at our respective institutions (London South Bank University, City University London and Nottingham University), as well as colleagues at the universities of Bologna, Guyana, Oxford, Sussex and University of the West Indies (at Cave Hill, Barbados and Mona, Jamaica), who provided homes for us as well as sound advice. We thank Professor Rosalind Edwards and Professor Janet Holland, for their support and leadership of the Families & Social Capital ESRC Research Group as well as other members of the Ethnicity Strand of this Group at London South Bank University; the Economic and Social Research Council (ESRC) for financial support in undertaking this work; referees of our proposal to Routledge; our editors at Routledge, who have not only been forgiving but have been generous and very understanding; and members of our Advisory Group and virtual network advisory group in the United States, Continental Europe, Australia and elsewhere.

In particular, we wish to thank the very many individuals in families and communities in Britain, the Caribbean, Italy, India and elsewhere who shared intimate details about their private lives with us.

Professor Ralph Grillo has consistently been an endless source of support, and we are delighted to be again in his debt for kindly providing us with a preface to this book.

An undertaking of this kind makes considerable demands on family life. We therefore thank our respective family members across the generations, from those who are moving into 'the vale of years' to those who – during the course of our work – sprung forth like lions, brightening our relationships and developing our collective resources.

Preface

International migration is changing the social and cultural composition of contemporary societies, sometimes posing difficult questions about living with difference and diversity. Two features of that migration have attracted the attention of policymakers and practitioners as well as social scientists. While many migrants still come to work in countries such as the UK on a temporary basis, others have long since settled down, and established a wide range of community institutions. One consequence is that the population of migrant or refugee origin is now substantially a family population, with implications for housing, health and educational systems in receiving countries which in varying degrees have been implementing neoliberal economic and social agendas, running down provision for welfare.

Settlement, however, did not mean that those who originally came as migrants or refugees abandoned all ties to countries of origin. Although many so-called migrants are long-term settlers, or have been born and brought up in receiving countries, their links with sending countries have not necessarily diminished, and a huge amount of literature over the last decade has explored the way in which individuals, households, families and whole communities find themselves with stakes in interconnected worlds, widely separated spatially, which they try to maintain simultaneously. They live, as we say, 'multi-sited' lives. While this phenomenon is not new, by the twenty-first century the revolution in information and communication technologies, and cheap international air travel, enabled millions of people to be 'doubly engaged', as Valentina Mazzucato has called it, 'here' and 'there'. At the same time, neither transnationalism nor globalization (of which it is part) have led to the withering away of the nation-state. Indeed, transnational life, with households sometimes scattered across the globe, may oblige family members to engage with, and be affected by, a multiplicity of states and state systems.

One of the virtues of the present volume is that the authors through their research have brought together these big themes (as has begun to happen in a limited number of other studies), and linked them through some key analytical and theoretical concepts in the social sciences, notably 'identity' and 'social capital'. This proves to be a powerful way of investigating both the relationship between families of migrant origin and the society in which they have settled, and relations within those families across gender and generation.

A further strength of this volume is its comparative focus. The research on which the book is based deals comparatively with several minorities present in the UK including people of African–Caribbean, Italian and South Asian origin. Many ethnic and racial studies are content to report in very general terms about migrants or ethnic minorities, or alternatively provide an in-depth account of particular populations or 'communities' in relative isolation. While such studies are valuable, the significance of their findings may only emerge in comparing their trajectories with those of others. Thus, one conclusion of the present study, is that the:

> children and grandchildren of Caribbean and Italian migrants are carving out new identities for themselves which combine and incorporate their connections with the Caribbean and Italian Diaspora, their lives in UK and continued links to the familial homeland.

In this case the trajectories appear to be similar; in others, perhaps in respect of 'mixed' partnerships for example, they may not be. Unravelling such complexities poses a considerable challenge to the social sciences. Secondly, although the book is principally concerned with the UK and presents an in-depth account of its subject in that context, the authors are fully aware of studies elsewhere and this allows them to embed their research in wide-ranging international literature, and enables the reader to begin to draw some conclusions about similarities and differences between the UK and other countries experiencing the same phenomena.

By enlarging the scope of ethnic and racial studies in these ways, the research breaks through some of the self-imposed boundaries that have long characterised work in this field in the UK. As such, it represents a notable, highly innovative and ethnographically rich contribution to a topic of considerable public importance.

Ralph Grillo,
Professor Emeritus, Anthropology,
University of Sussex
April 2009

Part I
Some general questions

1   Theorizing transnational families

Introduction

This book is about one of the most exciting developments in the related fields of human and social studies – transnational families. These families have extensive living links across national boundaries, and there is increasing interest in this relatively new phenomenon as crucial social, economic and political aspects of globalization. Members of these families and their wider kinship groups also pose questions about the crossing of boundaries other than the nation-state, such as those of 'race', ethnicity, gender and sexuality, and generation. The subject or problematic of transnational families, therefore, raises intriguing or provocative questions about such matters as migration, identities, communities, resources and relationships in the contemporary world. Arguably, the socially diverse post-imperial society emerging in Britain is one of the most dynamic in which these changes are taking place, and this book is about families in Britain with extensive transnational links across the globe, particularly the Caribbean and Italy. The book is the product of a multidisciplinary collaboration among researchers from the disciplines in the humanities and social studies,[1] with interests in families, migration, ethnic and racial identities, and other related issues.

It is, therefore, important that in this opening chapter we set out our main aims and explain the organization of this exploratory work of collaboration in what is becoming an important field of comparative study. It is equally important to make clear from the outset the central concept holding this work together. In the following chapter we examine some key concepts – particularly the concepts of ethnic and racial identities, communities, and social capital – and throughout the book we draw upon other concepts that help us to analyse our data and explain our arguments. But at this point of our discussion it is appropriate to say what we understand by the concept of 'transnational families', and how we want to deploy it throughout the book.

The transnational family phenomenon

The first thing to note about studies of transnational families is that although the different bodies of literature in which they appear are quite considerable and are growing (see, for example, Fouron and Schiller 2001; Bashi 2007; Goulbourne and Chamberlain 2001; Grillo 2008) there is still a relative dearth of theoretical discussion of the concept itself. While the idea of transnational families surfaces in debates about a wide range of phenomena which transcend the nation-state – such as globalization, migration, communication, travel, diasporas and cosmo-politanism – the concept is generally taken for granted or obvious, assumed to be unproblematic, and therefore readily understood. It is assumed that the concept is a straightforward description of families whose members live in different countries but manage to continue to keep in touch with each other. Of course, to a large extent this is indeed the case. But left in this way the concept is of little analytical use because it remains too large, too porous, and therefore too vague; the phenomena that we perhaps intuitively sense to be new remain elusive or slippery.

For example, recent studies focusing on Asian and Caribbean families in Britain and continuing contacts with their 'homelands' strongly reflects this assumption. Included in this body of work are some of our own (see for example, Goulbourne and Chamberlain 2001; Reynolds 2001; Goulbourne 2002) and the works of others (Western 1992; Bauer and Thompson 2006; Chamberlain 2006). Pnina Werbner's work (2002) on Pakistanis in Manchester as well as Katy Gardner's (2002) on Sylhetis in London are also cases in point. However, to be fair, these writers' concerns were more about specific recent immigrant communities and their links with their homelands than with the concept of transnational families; while their works suggest links between families and transnational experiences, this link – irrespective of what it may be – is not the primary subject of concern. These researchers' attention focused on the institution of the family dispersed across national boundaries within the context of migration, but the specificity of the transnational experience as applied to families as a problem of theory has been of less explicit concern.

From a different perspective Jaipaul Roopnarine and Uwe Gielen's work (2005) is a good illustration of studying families in a range of cultural contexts, without broaching the problematic of transnational families. This quite comprehensive and valuable collection ranges across the globe, with specific attention to families in different cultures. The editors and three contributors pull together a number of themes of general concern about 'the family' in modern societies, but the rest of the collection focuses on culturally embedded particular situations.

These, like other works, have not seen the transnational family experience as theoretically problematic, and have not therefore sought to set out the possible theoretical issues – origins, development and distinctive characteristics – that may be involved in accounting for the phenomenon of transnational families. What, however, has been achieved by the work of scholars generally concerned about the phenomenon is the provision of an overall context for a more rigorous approach to the notion of transnational families in the age of globalization. Arguably, there is something of an emerging field of study drawing on a number of academic disciplines and social issues centred on families across boundaries and scattered across sometimes vast physical distances. As a result of the attention given to these developments, we are coming to see that studies about migration, return and circular migration patterns, remittances, investments and diasporas, are all closely related to the problematic of transnational families and the different national communities or communal spaces that families straddle.

But, while there is not yet a concerted effort focusing on developing a theory of transnational families – where the fields of family studies and transnationalism are rigorously brought together – there is at least one notable exception to this general observation. This is Deborah Bryceson and Ulla Vuorela's introductory essay to their edited work entitled *The Transnational Family: New European Frontiers and Global Networks* (Bryceson and Vuorela 2002). Drawing on an impressive set of scholarship in related fields, their introduction – 'Transnational families in the twenty-first century' – breaks new ground by sharply focusing on the overall problematic of transnational families. In addition to this thoughtful and helpful introduction, this collection contains essays that seriously attempt to address the transnational experiences of families. In particular, Vuorela's 'Transnational families: imagined and real communities' picks up on the concept of communities drawing on Benedict Anderson's (2006) influential notion of the 'imagined' community created by nationalists – a matter of relevance to our explanation of communities in the next chapter. For now, we want to highlight three key aspects of Bryceson and Vuorela's essay that are highly relevant to the themes in this book.

First, we firmly agree with their view that the proper context for the study of transnational families is constituted by such factors as the renewed interest in and reformulation of the notion of diasporas, the fact of globalization, and the experiences of large-scale migration. As Bryceson and Vuorela point out, the works of scholars such as Avtar Brah (1996) and Robin Cohen (1996, 2008) are highly relevant here, and there are others whose works are highly relevant to the search for understanding in what may be an emerging multidisciplinary field (see, for example, Gardner and Grillo 2002; Goulbourne 2002; Zontini 2004b; Reynolds 2005; Bauer and Thompson 2006).

However, more so than Bryceson and Vuorela, we want to insist that transnational families and these contextual developments are to be understood within a world of nation-states. In subsequent chapters, particularly in Chapter 4, we explain and develop this point by showing the importance of these key parameters for the study of the transnational experiences for family units and their individual members in the contemporary world.

Second, Bryceson and Vuorela hinted that the experience of transnational families is not new, but we would like to assert this point more strongly. Bryceson and Vuorela correctly stress the movements of elites such as intellectuals and business people as well as colonial rulers and administrators representing transnational families before what is described as the postmodern age. We would add though that missionaries and teachers, and adventurers and travellers in Europe's empires abroad, contributed to the general context of the formation of transnational families over the last three or more centuries. This imperial type of transnationalism gave rise to such situations as the development of boarding schools, long-distance living and consciousness, and senses of belongingness irrespective of physical space. Similarly, in pre-modern Europe, feudal landlords and members of their retinue with lands in different parts of the Continent and adjacent islands constituted the basis for transnational family experiences in so far as there were multiple and overlapping loyalties and jurisdictions.

Beyond Bryceson and Vuorela, we want to stress that in late modernity the transnational experience has become commonplace for families irrespective of social class, although, as Ralph Grillo (2008) reminds us, social class does shape how transnationalism is experienced. The transnational experience has become part of the lives of working-class people as well as well-heeled middle-class families in society. While there has long been the movement of labour across national boundaries – through force of economic necessity, natural disasters or political repression – it is the growth of what Antony Giddens (2001) correctly called the world's first truly global society that has enabled this situation to become reality for ordinary, non-elite, families. The families whose experiences form the basis of our book are of this kind, and any acceptable theory of transnational families must incorporate the simple fact of the generalization of their experience in the contemporary world.

Third, in addition to the context, there are the elements of transnational family experiences to be considered and, again, Bryceson and Vuorela correctly highlighted a number of these. They pointed to three important categories: first, issues pertaining to care in old age; second, matters of identity (national, ethnic, belongingness); and third, the search for security and opportunity (political, economic, etc.). These are correctly seen as factors spawning transnational families, and these are the substance with which many scholars of the transnational experience are variously concerned (Glick-Schiller 1997; Baldassar 2001; Parreñas 2001; Christou 2002; Bauböck 2003; Levitt and de la Delera 2003; Gardner 2006; Beck-Gernsheim 2007; Levitt and Jaworsky 2007).

It may be suggested, however, that Bryceson and Vuorela perhaps underestimated the importance of identity and belongingness as crucial elements driving the motor of transnational family experiences. This underestimation may be seen particularly with regard to generation (youth and the aged), gender and sexuality, nationality and territory. We assert that these are vitally important elements in the engine that motors the phenomenon of transnational families as a norm in modern and contemporary societies.

Finally, while it is relevant to draw on Anderson's notion of 'imagined' communities (as Bryceson and Vuorela do) to describe transnational families, attempts to use this concept to understand the complex experiences of transnational families must be carefully applied or managed. After all, Anderson's thesis starts from the observation that it is difficult for the individual actually to have direct experience of the large collectivity described as 'the nation'. Though spatially dispersed across terrains and jurisdictions, families are small, discrete, units whereas nations are aggregate units. These differences are not trivial; they are fundamental to the understandings we seek to bring to the general context or framework of human interactions and social structures and will be returned to from time to time in our analysis.

Of particular importance in Bryceson and Vuorela's formulation of the problem are two key concepts that they offer to help us better understand the transnational experiences of families – what they call 'frontiering' and 'relativizing'. They employ the notion of 'frontiering'

> to denote the ways and means transnational family members use to create familial space and network ties in terrain where affinal connections are relatively sparse.
>
> (Bryceson and Vuorela 2002: 11)

They argue that this notion is preferable to that of 'negotiation' that has been widely used in the social sciences when discussing issues of identity. The concept of 'relativizing', on the other hand, refers 'to the variety of ways individuals establish, maintain and curtail relational ties with specific family members' (ibid.: 14). While the first of these concepts is easy enough to grasp, the second is more elusive, and it is not always clear how the one differs from the other. However, it is possible to understand 'frontiering' as referring to a family's relationship with others within a society in which the family has recently arrived from elsewhere, while 'relativizing' may be understood to refer 'back' to where the family originated.

Nonetheless, these are creative and suggestive notions. They can serve to link the past and the future, and irrespective of their strengths or weaknesses, the important point is that they are offered by Bryceson and Vuorela to kick-start a more crisp or robust theoretical approach to the problematic of transnational families. However, while we draw on Bryceson and Vuorela's work, we hope that our approach to the problematic of transnational families is both more nuanced and more loose or flexible than their definitions appear to suggest. We therefore draw attention to a number of specific points which bear out our differences to the question of the problematic of transnational families.

First, the central concepts of 'frontiering' and 'relativizing' may be too rigid or mechanical to be very helpful in describing the experiences of the transnational families whose stories of their collective and individual lives are the subject of this book. While these concepts may be flexible enough to take into account the fact that transnational families are dynamic and are agencies of change, they do not appear to be able satisfactorily to grapple with another fact – namely, that change occurs at both polar points of these families' experiences. This is so for several reasons. For example, 'back' in the homeland significant changes occur after a family's departure for the 'frontier', and at this point of arrival change occurs not only to the new arrivants but also to the indigenous or historic families and communities. There appear to be many wheels within wheels simultaneously turning; when this turning is in the same direction we are wont to see this as descriptive of transnationalism; when they turn in different directions they are omitted from the transnational narrative.

In addition, the world in which transnational families have to deal is likely to be more complex than that presented by the bipolar situation depicted. Families with functional transnational links tend to have scions or individual members scattered in more than two countries, suggesting that a nuanced definition of transnational families is necessarily more complex than Bryceson and Vuorela suggest. They define the transnational family thus:

> families that live some or most of the time separated from each other, yet
> hold together and create something that can be seen as a feeling of collective
> welfare and unity, namely, 'familyhood', even across national borders
>
> (Bryceson and Vuorela 2002: 3)

This is all too vague and open. Families within the same nation-state could easily come within this definition: families in large societies such as China or India may be distributed across several boundaries as may families in relatively small but highly socially mobile, unified but densely populated societies as Britain. As noted earlier, it is clear that the understanding that Bryceson and Vuorela brings to the discussion of the transnational family transcends the rather vague definition they themselves offer. But they are aware of the multiple factors that condition the context of transnational families, and this is a vitally important aspect of their contribution to the enterprise of understanding contemporary transnational families.

Second, time is as necessary to the definition of transnational families as is spatial distribution, and it is difficult to see how the notion of 'frontiering' helps us to capture this dimension of these families' lives and consciousness over time. While 'frontiering' may be highly suggestive of the experiences of immigrant families and their immediate offspring and even the families these offspring create, the concept does not account for subsequent developments. After two or more generations, it hardly makes sense to speak of these families' experiences as 'frontiering', even though there may still be cases of strong transnational links. After all, in the late nineteenth century one aspect of Frederick Turner's notion of 'the frontier' in American history was that it continued to expand (westward) in what became the USA; the US frontier kept being pushed forward to the Pacific and indeed eventually into the ocean itself in Hawaii. In contrast, the Roman frontier (the key model that Bryceson and Vuerola use) was a sharper divide between 'civilized' Romans and 'barbarian' others, particularly after the first emperor, Augustus, established boundaries of the empire in Europe, Africa and Asia. In short, the notion of 'frontiering' – like that of 'pioneers' that is entering the literature on migration and settlement – developed from well-established historical experiences is useful but only at the time of contact; it is less useful as time moves on, and the rejection by Bryceson and Vuorela of the notion of 'negotiation' to indicate identity formation may therefore be premature. We suggest that the notion of 'negotiation', which we will use from time to time in this book, contains something of the flexibility we seek to bring to the analysis of transnational families, as explained in the next chapter.

In concluding this section of our discussion, it is important to stress that Bryceson and Vuorela's contribution signals the need to problematize or seek some general overview of the notion of the transnational family and they have taken us beyond the largely descriptive or 'taken for granted' understanding of this generalized aspect of people's lived experience in an age of globalization. It may now be useful briefly to summarize or itemize some of the features we think would be necessary to include in a generalized theory of transnational families and which will be carried forward in the discussion in the rest of this book.

Boundaries of transnational families

First, while it is of central importance to recognize the jurisdictional context of the nation-state as a given of the transnational families experience, it is equally relevant to recognize the cultural worlds that these families occupy. In other words, the processes of globalization enable families to maintain links across national boundaries, across cultural divides and across spatial distances. It is obvious that with mass migration across national boundaries, the transnational experience is becoming common and open to families almost everywhere. Advances in communication technology – particularly the mobile phone, the Internet, inexpensive or affordable flights and digital cameras – have provided families with the means for keeping in close touch across vast spaces. Transnational families give substance to what Manuel Castells (2000) dubbed 'the network society', and this in turn minimizes the importance of physical distance and proximity. Migration and distance, therefore, no longer necessarily entail total loss of contact between family members or even scions of families and wider kinship networks. Transnational families may, therefore, be said to reflect modernity's increasing push against the barriers of nature.

Second, it must be stressed that the networks formed by families across national boundaries is a crucial aspect of globalization because it is not just a matter of families divided across two nation-states. Transnational families generally tend to be scattered across several nation-states, and this shows a world in which ordinary people are able relatively freely to negotiate physical, social and cultural spaces to suit their felt or perceived needs, wants or aspirations. In this context, different kinds of movements of families come into play. The obvious cases are, of course, return and circular migrations. The latter is the easier to understand: individuals and families move from A to B to C locations across national boundaries, and either whole families or individual members may repeatedly traverse or negotiate these routes.

But what has been described as return migration is becoming a complex matter. For example, sometimes the 'returnee' is not actually a 'returnee' (Thomas-Hope 2009): such a person or persons may in truth be a *bona fide* returnee, that is, a person who migrated from country A to country B and returns to country A. Migrants may reassemble their existing families or create new ones, or participate in both processes. But either migrants themselves or, more likely, their offspring, beget new families and some of these new members are from other communities. This is particularly so in the British case, because of the high propensity of people from different racial and ethnic communities in Britain to marry or establish sexual and family partnerships with individuals outside their own groups. This crossing of racial and ethnic boundaries at the most intimate level of social life is spawning a literature around what some researchers call 'mixed' families (Bennington 1996; Callabero *et al.* 2008; Haritaworn 2009). This is expanding the transnational dimension of such families. The 'return' to a homeland may therefore be to a diverse range of regions and countries in the world where spouses and offspring follow one or more individuals sharing living arrangements within a family or a household.

Sometimes the 'return' is to a place in which the 'returnee' was not born nor ever lived, but which he or she may have visited as a tourist or traveller to meet other family members (Abenaty 2000). Indeed, the 'homeland' can be a place where family members have had no direct, personal, experience, but a place about which families develop myths of belongingness (Goulbourne 2002; Potter *et al*. 2005; Reynolds 2008). Of course, this is not uncommon in any particular country where internal migration or movement effects a dispersal of families. This becomes more interesting when the 'home' is a far away place, as we will see in later chapters of this book. In either case, a sense of physical place almost invariably plays a significant role in the shared memories of collective identities of our family units.

Third, several important things arise from this situation of families having another actual or imaginary home away from where they may lead their day-to-day lives. In the first instance, there is the potential for the nationalist demand for total commitment to a particular nation-state to be undermined. This need not be subversive in a political sense, but can force the issue of having multiple loyalties and commitments becoming more widely acceptable and seen to be normal. Offspring may be courted by governments in the parental 'homeland' for general support such as financial investment, votes or simply general association, and this may be of mutual benefits, particularly for small and poorer nation-states and for marginalized new minorities in dominant historic populations. This is what Alejandro Portes and his colleagues call transnationalism from above (Portes *et al*. 1999; Portes 2001).

Figure 1 below illustrates the general relationships or concerns of transnational families, and points to the various matters that such families are likely to be concerned about. Following Portes and his colleagues as well as Thomas Faist (2000), we construct these relationships or concerns in this manner in order to suggest the kinds of distinctions that may be made about matters that are deemed transnational: the broadly economic, the political and the socio-cultural. In this book, we focus on two sets of these relationships: broadly cultural matters, and care and provision issues. While we focus less directly on the broadly political and economic matters, as represented on the diagram, our analyses are intertwined from time to time with the economic and the political, and in any event there are implications in both directions. In general, the point of this construct is to illustrate the regions or areas of transnationalism that are subjects for the analysis of transnational families, not the coverage of this book.

Crucially, Portes and his colleagues (Portes *et al*. 1999) insist that the individual social actor should be the starting point or the proper unit or object of the analysis of transnationalism, and that we should distinguish this individual actor from institutions (parties, corporations, etc.). While Bryceson and Vuorela do not insist on this point, we wish to stress that the family may be a more fitting unit for the proper analysis of the social forces we grapple to come to terms with when we talk about the socio-cultural dimension of transnationalism. Portes' transnational individual is embedded within the family. Such an individual originates, continues along the road of life, and sees their social being within the context of family of birth and family of creation scattered across physical spaces and memorial times. For our individual, the points of departure and arrival, like the points of settlement and

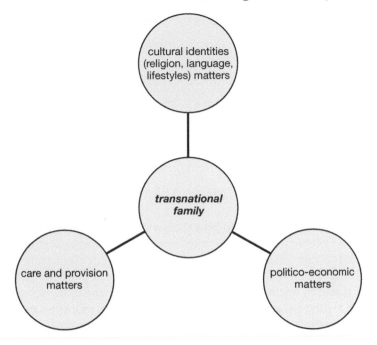

Figure 1 Transnational families' connections and concerns.

return, are located or buried within the bosom of the family. Arguably, therefore, the institution of the family and the various social practices associated with it, may be the best social space from where to explicate the problems of transnationalism with which scholars of this phenomenon have grappled over the last two decades or so. We do not wish to make such a strong and unqualified claim. But we do wish to assert that the social practices we collectively describe as the family is a crucial location for understanding a novel or original social phenomenon – this is where ordinary people lead lives that transcend the boundaries of the nation-state, and potentially threaten other social and cultural boundaries set by race, ethnicity, and so forth. Figure 2 suggests this complex set of relationships, interactions, disruptions and potential for change when different groups of people and families meet; they undermine some boundaries while maintaining others.

Portes and his colleagues correctly argue that not everything that encompasses the experiences of migrants should be taken to be elements of transnationalism. This too should be carried over to our consideration of transnational families: there are, for example, individuals and families who wish to distance themselves from their real and imagined pasts, and who resist calls to be members of the transnational collectivity. Integration into the society of arrival may be their main concern, and while this can also be coupled with problems 'back home', it need not be so. The possibility of absorption into the society of arrival may be the main objective of some groups, and continuing links with the homeland may take a very low priority or be totally rejected.

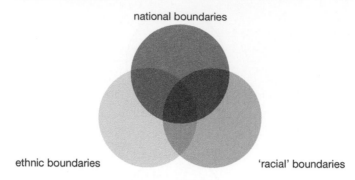

national boundaries

ethnic boundaries   'racial' boundaries

Figure 2 Cross-boundaries of the transnational family.

Finally, contrary to Portes and his colleagues, we do not define transnationals as only those people who engage in activities 'that require a regular and sustained social contacts over time across national borders for their implementation' (Portes *et al.* 1999: 219). Physical movements or the exchange of goods are not the only types of practices discussed in this book. Rather, we tend more to embrace the 'social field' perspective of Nina Glick-Schiller (2004: 457) whereby 'transnational social fields include individuals who have never themselves crossed borders but who are linked through social relations to people in distant and perhaps disparate locations'.

It must now be clear that the main aim of this book is to provide a plausible account of transnational family lives that are becoming more commonplace in a globalized world. In our account, such lives are bounded by multiple and overlapping identities as revealed or articulated in a range of social practices in everyday life as expressed in the narratives of ordinary people. These include ethnic and racial, gender and generational identities as well as what increasingly is being thought of as individuality or individual identity as reflected through the freedom individuals exercise in defining themselves. In the following chapter we spend some time explaining our understandings of these identities, each of which are highly contested and reflect not only the state of social studies but also the concerns of the general public and the policy world. For now, the meanings of these identities are taken for granted or set aside so as to allow us carefully to explain the general tenor of the book.

We utilize the concepts of 'bonding', 'bridging' and 'linking' social capital (Edwards *et al.* 2003; Goulbourne and Solomos 2003; Reynolds 2004; Zontini 2004b; Mand 2006) to understand how families scattered across the boundaries of nation-states manage to maintain close and meaningful links. Our examination concentrates on the lived experiences of three fairly distinct racio-ethnic communities, and our starting point is Britain. However, the overall work is set within the transnational contexts of family and community links from Britain to the Caribbean and to Italy, but we are also aware of other relevant experiences, such as the Greeks and South Asians in Britain. Drawing on the sizeable extant bodies of literature about racial and ethnic identities, social capital, migration and transnationalism, we argue that while social capital theory can be fruitfully utilized to enhance understanding of how families manage to maintain identities, give and receive support, the concept must be used iteratively rather than prescriptively. Based on our comparative research, our somewhat sceptical approach enables us to explore the strengths and weaknesses of the concept of social capital as is explained in the next chapter.

Our approach also helps us to combine insights emerging from different disciplines concerned with transnational families as a major feature of globalization and modernity. While there is much to be learnt from the many common features that transnational families share, each transnational family and kinship network must be understood in their own terms or contexts. The notion of transnational families does not therefore replace, but rather builds upon, the work of scholars and researchers who have explained the dynamics of families in and across different cultural and national contexts. This new dimension of the wider transnational experience may represent a major means of subverting or transforming the close-knit integrity of the nation-state as the sole basis of political legitimacy and social action.

Organization of the book

The book is divided into two parts: in this first part we continue to discuss some major issues of theory and method, such as the concepts and utility of 'social capital', 'community across national boundaries', and 'changing family forms' as well as tackle the abiding problems of how we conduct multidisciplinary and comparative research, and the relevance of this approach within a transnational world. This part of the book enables us to establish connections with discussions taking place outside the scope of our empirical research. In Part II we pick up on a number of common themes and issues that emerged from our interviews of transnational families.

Chapter 2 sets out a critical account of discussions about the issues involved in the often disjointed, though generally assumed to be closely related, discourses about families, ethnic identities and communities. There is a range of issues and voices involved here, and we critically dissect some of these, and locate our comparative research into these debates. The chapter briefly describes the meanings of some important concepts that run throughout the book: first, ethnic and 'racial' identities and categories; social capital; and families and communities. Second, the chapter explores the concept and utility of social capital as funnelled through (a) identities and values (b) trust and reciprocity and (c) caring for and about members of families and communities

It is very important to set out, and reflect upon, the methodological problems we encountered when conducting research across national, ethnic and racial boundaries. The problems and opportunities, or the limitations and strengths, of collaborative research in social studies are therefore discussed in Chapter 3. Involved here are the complexity of how individuals, families, and communities perceive, utilize and reproduce their ethnicities as social capital; the kinds of changes that occur within families as a result of ethnic plurality or mixing in a multicultural society; explaining how ethnicity as social capital is reproduced within the discrete domains of families and kinship relationships across national boundaries; and consideration of the theoretical implications for our understanding of social capital and social change.

Chapter 4 rounds off the overall setting or context for the substantive discussions that follow in the second part of this book. The chapter focuses on the politics of migration and issues about diversity and discrimination that have characterized important aspects of public concerns in Britain since at least the late 1950s.

The chapters in the second part of the book discuss specific issues about transnational families and social capital in practice (bonding, bridging, linking), and similarities and differences in the Caribbean and Italian communities in Britain. These discussions begin in Chapter 5, which examines the settlements of migrants and their offspring by outlining where families with Caribbean and Italian backgrounds chose to settle in Britain and where their communities sprung up; the development of friendships beyond ethnic and racial boundaries; and the significance of the physical location as an aspect of identity-building.

Chapter 6 is concerned with family members' needs and provision of support across borders. We explore how transnational families see the need to provide material and emotional supports to members of the kinship network; how these arrangements are said to be reciprocated around issues demanding 'caring about' and 'caring for' each other. We emphasize aspects of continuities in values and social practices as illustrations of the positive side of the utilization or mobilization of family and community social capital in Chapter 7. Some of the negative features of close-knit, tightly bonded families and communities are explored in Chapter 8. For example, the chapter analyses the *angst* experienced by some of those who are described by many writers as 'second' and 'third' generations – a notion that we reject because of its factual inaccuracy and its political implications and instead refer to migrants and their offspring.

The question of 'return to the source', 'the homeland' or 'back home' is an abiding and crucial aspect of the immigrant's story or narrative of identities. Chapter 9 explores this phenomenon and shows how it is a highly complex matter, but one that illustrates the immigrant's and their offspring's relationships with both the new society of settlement and the earlier point of departure. Again, this is currently a crucial issue in much political and policy discourses in Britain, and the chapter seeks to contextualize the findings from our research. We explore the patterns of 'return' of immigrants to Britain from our regional and national sites; the ways in which 'immigrant communities' and families invest (emotionally and otherwise) in 'homelands', as well as how some 'homelands' now provide material supports for people abroad who are seen as 'belonging', and can therefore be claimed. Chapter 10 describes family formation across the boundaries of racial and ethnic identities. In the final chapter we make some suggestions about possible areas for future discussion and research, as well as areas for policy considerations. The chapter seeks to encourage similar comparative research, and point to the value of this for the building of a post-imperial Britain and a globalized world that are still in the making. We thereby return to the central questions discussed in Part I of the book, and we draw out some policy and research implications of our work.

Conclusion

In this chapter we have set out to do two things. First, we have sought to outline how we intend to conduct our discussion of one of the crucial subjects of our time – the experience of families cast across national as well as a number of other boundaries and who are therefore being described as transnational families. Second, we have set out what have been our aims and objectives in embarking on this collaborative venture. Both these objectives will be further developed in the chapters that follow in this first part of the book. The next step, therefore, is to more fully enter into the questions that our subject and assertions raise, and it is to these that we now turn.

Note

1   The book emerges from our work as part of the Ethnicity Strand of the Families and Social Capital Economic and Social Research Council (ESRC) Research Group from 2002. The Group's work consisted of three interrelated strands about families in contemporary Britain, and the Strand's work represents one of the most sustained attempts to carry out empirical research on transnational families in Britain.

2 Social capital joins the trinity

Families, ethnicities, communities

Introduction

In this chapter we explore the main concepts that are essential to our analysis of transnational families – ethnic and related identities, communities and social capital. These concepts are central to issues that have been at the heart of significant debates throughout the social sciences. In this book, as in our research, our aim has been and remains to engage with these concepts in relation to transnational families and their experiences in British society, in their countries of origin and in the wider globalized social and cultural environments. At the starting point of our research the issue of social capital was seen by many as a key issue that the social sciences had to address, particularly in relation to popular concerns about a breakdown in social cohesion and radical changes in the role of the family in contemporary societies. At the same time there was particular concern about the interface between this question and the reality that societies such as that in Britain were becoming increasingly multicultural in both their demographic composition and emerging family forms.

These have been central to academic and popular as well as political and policy concerns over the last decade and are likely to continue to be at the forefront of social and political unease and discussion in Britain and elsewhere for the foreseeable future. After all, despite the onslaught on, and the scepticism about, the ideals or aspirations and policy of multiculturalism, Britain is generally thought to exhibit one of the richest or generous societies, exhibiting a variety of communities as reflected in family types, traditions and close and continuing links with extensive kinship networks originating in, and extending to, a number of other European countries, Africa, the Caribbean and Asia. These are parts of the world with which, historically, Britain had, and continues to have, close links and, as we will see in Chapter 3, these are also the regions from which our samples of transnational families are drawn.

While, therefore, Chapter 4 situates transnational families within the general context of migration, the nation-state and globalization, this chapter is organized around our understandings of, first, families and communities; second, identities; and third, the question of whether and how the concept of social capital is helpful in understanding the nexus of relationships and resources that family and community life involve across national boundaries in our global age.

Families and communities

Traditionally, the institution of the family was generally thought to be the basic unit of a social system with the function of providing for the biological and social reproduction of human society. Spinning outward from the family core (whether nuclear or extended) is the kinship group, which is a series of networks connected through biological but equally importantly through social and legal sanctions (through such acts as marriage, and such players or agencies as in-laws). While there may be general agreement with this broad definition, the last two decades or so have witnessed a growing dissatisfaction with what we assume constitutes the institution of the family. For example, it has been suggested that the inner nucleus of the traditional family constituted through the partnership/marriage of two adults, used to be represented as 'me + you' (a merger in which both entities lose their autonomy or separate identities); today the representation takes the form of 'me+you+us' – three fairly distinct entities (Furstenberg 2005). This trinity that is displacing the traditionally fused duo gives recognition to the atomization or individualization of intimate relationships (see, for example, Giddens 1992; Bauman 1996; Beck and Beck-Gersheim 2002; also, Smart and Shipman 2004). Irrespective of these changes, two points may be noted here: first, families are generally located within the context of wider kinship networks; and, second, these in turn are structured and operate within communities located in specific physical spaces, and/or scattered across unconnected territories, such as with transnational families (see, for example, Goulbourne and Chamberlain 2001; Goulbourne 2002; Bryceson and Vuorela 2002), as we will see in the following chapter.

There are therefore several new factors about family life or living arrangements to be taken into account. In the first place, it is increasingly asserted that 'family' may be constituted without there necessarily being blood parentage or descent. The growth in the numbers of people who wish to adopt children is an obvious case in point, and they include gay and lesbian partners as well as heterosexual couples who (for one or more biological or social reasons) cannot have children of their own. Then there are those who would argue that friends may come to constitute closer and more meaningful relationships than family members connected by descent and or legal sanctions. Moreover, there have long been communities who have used the concept of family metaphorically to indicate close bonds through shared values, provision of mutual support and commitment, such as monks, nuns and other ascetic as well as secular sects.

In the main, however, the typologies of the families with backgrounds in the Caribbean, Asia, southern Europe, and other parts of the world fit more or less into what may be termed 'traditional'. But what is meant by 'traditional' needs to be explained with regard to Caribbean and Italian families on whom we focus in this book.

***

First, even though no study has specifically focused on British-Italian families, family relationships and the nature of 'the Italian family' are discussed in several studies and these are often explained as central characteristics of Italian ethnicity. In this literature, what seems to distinguish Italians both from other immigrant groups and from the majority population is the specific role and characteristics attributed to the family. According to Fortier (2000: 61), the literature on Italians in the UK associates the Italian family 'with "traditional" values that no longer have the same currency within the dominant "host" culture'. One example of this position is Colpi who describes the Italian family in the following way:

> The most important unit, basic to the way of life and the structure of the community, is the family. Although individualism is the mark of Italianism, the family is the very core of the Community ... While particularly important for the new immigrants, the family ethic nevertheless still holds considerable sway amongst the 'old' settlers and their descendants who are more family conscious than the population at large.
>
> (Colpi 1991: 191)

One problem with this literature is that it can inadvertently contribute to fixed and monolithic images of the Italian family. In spite of the commonality just described, there are important differences in the way authors interpret the role of 'the British-Italian family' which reflect the more complex nature and diversity of Italian families. For instance, whereas some seem to see British-Italian families as harmonious cooperative units, others note the power inequalities that divide them. Also, whereas for some, families are the basic units from which wider relations of cooperation and solidarity are built, for others they represent the limit of associative life and integration.

Thus, for Palmer (1977) and Colpi (1991), the strong reciprocal links between kin members explain the form and specificity of Italian migration. For Colpi, such links involve 'a process whereby families from particular villages or regions move to a new country or to a city, from which they instigate a "chain migration" by assisting their relatives to join them' (Colpi 1991: 19). Of course, Italian migration to Britain and elsewhere has taken other forms – such as recruitment schemes – but the mechanism of chain migration was the main way in which very many people from specific villages in Italy found their way to specific locations in Britain and other parts of the world.

Italian family values and norms have also been used to explain the particular insertion and success of Italians in the catering trade. It is believed that Italians have been able to open venues catering to the needs of fellow Italians – restaurants, cafés, ice-cream bars – because of the cohesion of their families. As Palmer (1977: 251) explained, 'their production is only made possible by the mobilization of family labour, with everyone working long hours'. Colpi (1991), stressed that Italians were successful in trading on their ethnicity, not only by selling 'ethnic' products but also by turning specific family values into economic success.

Earlier, Bottignolo (1985) perceived great strengths in how Italian families were able to maintain inter-generational cohesion. Like others, he saw British-Italian families as largely harmonious units. In his study of Italians in the Bristol area, he saw little inter-generational conflict and attributed the lack of such conflict and the tightness of family ties to the 'gratifying and qualifying environment of the immigrant family group' (1985: 196). He observed that

> Italian immigrants perceive the role of the family differently from the way English people do. In the Italian immigrant family, individual interests are merged in the general interest of the family group. All members put their efforts in the service of the family and when one starts thinking of getting out (usually by marrying) all the members of the family contribute in order to help him or her settle.
>
> (Bottignolo 1985: 194)

In his study of Calabrians in Bedford, Cavallaro (1981) also saw evidence of the continuation of Italian cultural values. Whereas Bottignolo saw the strength of British-Italian families in its 'gratifying and qualifying environment', for Cavallaro such strength is a result of the family's function as a 'buffer zone' between the individual and the inhospitable society in which the immigrants arrived (1981: 71). Cavallaro also acknowledged that the norms of reciprocity and solidarity that existed in the Calabrian nuclear family were based on relationships among members that were asymmetric. The father remained a powerful patriarch who had to be respected and be obeyed by his children, and Cavallaro noted how children were prevented from breaking away from the family by a sense of their debt of gratitude for the 'sacrifice' that their parents (especially the father) had made.

Bottignolo (1985: 78) noted that 'a variety of personal relations often over and above the kinship type' were of 'considerable importance' for Italian immigrants in Bristol. For Cavallaro (1981), however, solidarity and trust operated only within families. Even though he admitted that Calabrians were involved in activities of reciprocity, such as the exchange of produce from their allotments and help with repairing tasks, Cavallaro saw these forms of solidarity and trust as a declining resource. He thought that social relationships were becoming increasingly competitive, with the result that Calabrians were less willing to engage in exchanges outside their close-knit families. Similarly to the theme of 'amoral familism' found in the Italian literature on families, Cavallaro concluded that '[t]he compactness of the family microcosm, its size, the strong values of group cohesion, are obstacles against the birth and development of associations' (Cavallaro 1981: 115).

Whereas Bottignolo describes the lack of intergenerational conflict in Italian families, Colpi (1991) entitles one section of her book on Italians in the UK: 'Conflict'. In that section she describes the tensions over contrasting values that, during the 1960s and 1970s, started to emerge between parents and children. She notes how, during this time, the family was not a tightly knit economic unit any more, and women and children had gained considerable power vis-à-vis their father. Second-generation children: 'on the one hand strove to be independent and accepted by their English peers but, on the other, they had been molded to accept the wishes of their parents and desired to maintain the good name of their family' (Colpi 1991: 202).

Chistolini (1986) too, in her study of Italo-Scottish women, noted the latent conflicts between the values that young Scottish women of Italian origin learnt at school and those transmitted in their families. Both Colpi and Chistolini observed that these young people rarely rebelled openly against their parents. The reason for their acceptance of imposed norms and behaviour was, according to Colpi, not the result of harmonious family relations but the effect of very strict social control exercised by both family and community, especially in small cities such as Bedford where large groups of Italians settled.

Both Chistolini (1986) and Colpi (1991) identified diversity as an important aspect of Italian family life in Britain because of the different migration histories of people from different parts of Italy. Colpi differentiated between the old and the new Italian communities (pre- and post-1945 migration), whereas Chistolini distinguished between those families in which women migrated around the 1960s and migration since that decade. Both authors stressed common characteristics among Italian families. In Chistolini's view, women were generally responsible for creating and maintaining the cohesion, solidarity and unity of the family, and were involved in paid work outside the home. But their extra domestic activities were seen as supporting the family in their needs. The links across the generations were considered to be very strong, and when married offspring left the parental home, they settled nearby and maintained regular inter-household contacts with their kin. For Colpi (1991), offspring of migrant families tended to retain several of what she called 'traditional patterns', which included the separation of roles between husband and wife; strong relationships with same-sex kin; maintenance of face-to-face contact with immigrant parents; and reliance on the many services that the family network can offer. As Colpi observed,

> These include a considerable amount of financial help from both sets of parents in the early days of marriage, practical as well as economic help when the third generation emerges, and provision of certain ethnic items such as homemade wine, where the relevant manufacturing skills have not generally been acquired by the second generation.
>
> (Colpi 1991: 207)

More recent research on families of Italian backgrounds in Britain tends to focus on gender relations. Anne-Marie Fortier's *Migrant Belongings* (2000) and Azadeh Medaglia's *Patriarchal Structures and Ethnicity in the Italian Community in Britain* (2001) use different methodologies to examine and portray British-Italian women as resistant to change, as victims of patriarchal power, deeply religious and anchored to tradition. As Medaglia recognized, this depiction of the British situation sharply contrasts with the accounts of the changing and complex roles and positions of Italian women in Italy in recent years. It could be argued that immigrant communities retain traditional values and norms more strongly than the societies from where they originated, thus explaining a rigid conservation of a specific gender order. This is partly true. Both Fortier's and Medaglia's accounts very much resemble the kinds of descriptions that dominated much migration literature on Italians, but which has been subjected to feminist criticism. In such accounts, women were described as traditional, passive, subordinated to male migrants, and limited by their culture but Morokvasic (1983, 1984), Phizacklea (1983), and Bujis (1993), offer examples of the various and convincing critiques of this orthodoxy with regard to Britain. Similarly, studies on Italian women in other geographical and societal contexts (Vasta 1993; Gabaccia and Iacovetta 2002) point to the more complex role and position of Italian women in their families and immigrant communities. In subsequent chapters, we will draw upon and develop aspects of these perspectives of Italian families.

***

Second, with regard to families of Caribbean backgrounds in Britain, the dominant or main typology captured in representations of family and community life both in Britain and in the Caribbean is that of the lone mother, who is responsible for bringing up, nurturing and providing models of adult life for the child. Scholars in the Caribbean have variously suggested that this family type may be properly described as matrifocal (see, for example, Smith 1962a, 1962b; also Smith 1956, 2001), because the family and household are composed of adult females and dependent children, with men having a relationship with the women on a visiting (as distinct from residential) basis (see, Barrow 1996). While marriage and the nuclear unit are desirable, they tend to come well after child-rearing has commenced and can be quite late in the parents' relationship. Thus, in Britain for example, according to the 1991 national census (which introduced the so-called 'ethnic' question into the British national census), 51 per cent of African-Caribbean mothers were lone parents as compared with 14 per cent of mothers in the population as a whole, and less than 10 per cent in the South Asian communities. Some writers have argued that the living arrangements in these circumstances may be more complex than the notion of a matrifocal home suggests (see, for example, Smith 2001; Reynolds 2003). In both Britain and the Caribbean, therefore, the depiction of the family has long been a politically contested matter, with important implications for social policy. Three examples may be in order here.

First, the problem of parenting is often seen to centre on the poor level of fatherhood. Interestingly, there is comparatively little discussion about partnering issues, such as faithfulness, love and intimacy, other than perhaps in songs and popular discussion about black men's apparent preference for white women. There is, however, no question about the dedication of mothers to their offspring; indeed, in interviews about family life respondents tend to see their mothers in highly positive terms because of the care, love and guidance they provide for their children. Fathers, too, tend to express a sense of care about their children and tend not to see residential absence from the home of the mother and child as being necessarily a sign of a lack of care for the child. Additionally, it is sometimes suggested that the role of the biological father may be played by the presence of other males, such as uncles, grandfathers and older male siblings (Reynolds forthcoming 2009).

Whatever the case, the concern in Caribbean communities over the last decade has been such that there are now groups of men who join to provide positive role models to children, particularly boys, whose poor educational performance in the schools is sometimes blamed (perhaps not entirely inaccurately) on the absence of male models within the home.

Second, black families of Caribbean backgrounds in Britain have faced the problem of an absence of the extended family, that is, the household and kinship networks they would have relied upon in the Caribbean. This may be due to two factors: first, the migration patterns from the region; and, second, the tendency to return. In the first instance, many migrants who came to Britain between the late 1940s and the early 1960s, ended their working lives in the 1980s and 1990s. Many opted to realize their dream of returning to the Caribbean. While there may have been frequent visits in both directions across the Atlantic, the absence of grandparents means that families may now be in much the same position as they were during the years of immigration, with an absence of the extended members who can provide guidance, practical help for mothers who – more than mothers in other communities – are likely to be employed (see, for example, Barrow 1982; Owen 2001, 2006; Goulbourne 2002).

This leads to a third problematic issue: it may be hypothesized that black families of Caribbean backgrounds in Britain are not sites or agencies for the accumulation of resources that support upward social mobility. In nearly all social indices that measure social upward mobility – such as employment, residence and education – Caribbeans are situated at the lower ends, with many offspring doing less well than their parents and their grandparents, the original migrants. When combined with such factors as high levels of violence within neighbourhoods and communities, high levels of mental breakdown, and representation in prisons, it becomes clear that the family is both a crucial location for the individual as well as being an institution that cannot reasonably cope with all the problems brought to its doorstep.

With regard to the wider national British community, two general features of Caribbean families appear striking. While the social capital that has been described as 'bonding' – between all members of a group; between spouses; between fathers and offspring, etc. – may be seen as comparatively loose and fluid in Caribbean families, the kinds of social capital that theorists describe as 'linking' is very strong. Caribbean people have made links and built bridges across racial and ethnic boundaries particularly into the majority indigenous communities. While friendships, memberships of community, sporting organizations and so forth are important in this, of far greater significance has been the creation of families across these boundaries. Marriage, or perhaps more properly 'partnering', tends to be highly exogamous rather than endogamous, in contrast to most other communities. This, of course, raises tantalizing questions about the Caribbean family in Britain, such as whether it is adequately described as simply black, or, indeed, exclusively Caribbean.

Finally, these features combine to give Caribbean families in Britain the appearance of being precursors of some family types that are characteristic of late modernity. These include such features as single-parent, mother-centred or mother-led families; the looseness of the family structure and relationships; the porous boundaries emerging between family members across racial and ethnic identities; and perhaps most significantly, the growing tendency towards individualistic choice and autonomy. These features of late modernity involved serious risks along gender (men and women) and generational (children and the elderly) lines as traditional feelings of obligations and trust are presumed to erode. One lesson to be learnt from the Caribbean family model is that while these risks remain, and while they raise questions about state help for family members, they also show that care and obligations can be maintained across national boundaries (as will be shown in later chapters), and within loose, open and porous networks and social practices. These characteristics led to a preference (Goulbourne 2002) of the term 'living arrangements' when describing Caribbean families. The term suggests a broader social category than what has come to be a fairly narrow and focused construct of 'family'; it also suggests that the ways in which humans construct collective lives are not confined to the received forms of household and kinship networks inherited from the recent past, that is, the narrative of the nuclear family.

***

Necessarily, communities like families denote kinds of social relationships, but obviously communities are larger entities embracing any number of families. Additionally, both 'the family' and 'the community' have been claimed by a variety of groups, and this has opened up new understandings of the relationships involved in the family and in the community (see, for example, Plummer 2003; Weeks 2007). The notions of a family and a community may have to be 'imagined' in much the same way as Anderson (2006) suggested nations are imagined. To a degree, the imagination is called into play when bringing into focus members of the transnational family: they are scattered across space and time, and members do not necessarily share common day-to-day experiences, even though members do have some factors in common. In these circumstances, the wisdom garnered from classical sociology continues to have relevance. For example, Tonnies' (1955) distinction between *gemeinschaft* and *gesellschaft* may still be useful in making the necessary connections between families, kinship groups and communities. Where *gemeinschaft* represents communities based on living together (such as in the home, in the village or in a state or a country), *gesellschaft* represents communities based on legal contract or agreement with an identifiable aim in mind (such as in a marriage, in a business company, or in an interest group). Consistent with several nineteenth-century theorists, Tonnies was concerned to understand what made modern societies different from traditional societies, and identified the latter sense of community as being characteristic of modern societies. For example, when increasingly people use the word 'partner' to describe an intimate relationship between two individuals, it may be suggested that the vocabulary from *gesellschaft* is being used to convey a *gemeinschaft* relationship, and thereby undermining or questioning a dualism between 'the public' and 'the private' or the domestic domains of intimate and public relationships.

Today, we tend to be more cautious or nuanced in our assessments or characteri-
zations of different societies and try to avoid sharp dualities. Consequently, we may
be more inclined to take into account both the 'traditional' and the 'modern' senses
of community asserting themselves in intimate relationships, the acquisition and
sharing of resources. Of course, the simple dichotomies such as Tonnies' *gemeinschaft* and *gesellschaft*, or Émile Durkheim's 'mechanical' and 'organic', or Karl
Marx's pre-capitalist and capitalist as well as Max Weber's distinction between
'traditional' and 'modern' societies have usefully served what Weber called 'ideal
types' to help us better to understand transformative changes in human societies.
However, today we are perhaps better placed both to understand these mark-off
points as well as to see the often subtle intertwining of the past and the present,
between the traditional and the modern, and particularly the conflicts between the
forces and tensions involved in the interplay.

At this point it is necessary to ask the functionalist question about what families
and communities are for in society. We would suggest that both have at least four
key functions. With regard to families, it is generally assumed, first, that they are
the agency in which intimate relationships are realized; second, these generally lead
to reproduction of our species, that is, individuals like ourselves; third, this institution provides material and emotional resources and supports for members; fourth,
the family acts as a basic unit or agent of socialization of new members. Through
all four tasks the family serves to link individuals to the wider kinship group, and to
the wider community made up of yet more families and kinship networks – society.
The community to which families and individuals may feel that they belong or are
presumed by others to belong may be characterized by shared history, longevity
of residence, hardships and other trials of life, icons, language, religious and other
beliefs and values. The community will not only provide wider socialization of
members beyond the family, but will also give meaning to the 'imagined' wider
collectivity to which discrete groups and individuals are presumed to share certain
factors. The community also exerts restraints and constraints on individual and
group behaviour – as, following Durkheim, so many social analysts have emphasized. And the community equips members with such factors as the infrastructure
of language, values, and sometimes also provide the basic structure of day-to-day
life such as the means whereby individuals and families earn a living through the
work in which they participate.

Collective identities

The kinds of communities with which this chapter is concerned exhibit racial and
ethnic identities that are supposed to be distinct from the racial and ethnic identities
of the majority population. While this assumption represents one level of reality, at
another level this is a misrepresentation or distortion of the situation. Both racial
(meaning phenotypical differences, such as they are) and ethnic (cultural values,
traditions, customs, etc.) factors that distinguish South Asians, Caribbeans, and
the historic majority population of the country point to some obvious differences.
However, these apparently obvious differences also hide significant similarities and

overlappings of group identities. Of particular significance in the British context is the fact that over the last half of the twentieth century the entry, settlement and consolidation of new communities have not resulted in communities marked off by irreconcilable value systems and an absence of inter-racial mixing and mingling in terms of either of Tonnies' communities – that is, neither in living arrangements nor in formal, contractual relationships. Of course, the identities that Asians and Caribbeans in contemporary Britain answer to or express are new, although they have antecedents. Put simply, the notion of 'Asian' disappears in the sub-continent as does 'African Caribbean' in the Caribbean region, because these are largely British constructions – whether of a colonial kind as in East Africa with 'Asians' or within post-imperial island Britain, as with 'African Caribbeans'.

We want to emphasize a simple point here: we understand ethnicity to signify socio-cultural factors such as shared histories, memories, myths, customs, sentiments, beliefs and values. Of particular importance are religion and language. Indeed, the assertion of religion as a key ethnic defining factor has not only been more than noticeable in Britain over the last two decades, but it has also led some writers and commentators – confusingly – to treat religion as a factor transcending ethnic identity. It goes without saying that the combination of these factors or elements which may define an ethnic identity are subject to change, but at an aggregate societal level what is interesting about ethnic identity is its capacity for auto-maintenance, as well as its incorporation of a high degree of change without always destroying flagged particularistic characteristics. From this perspective, it is possible to recognize that identities evolve and change over time and space, while somehow taking along a combination of social elements. Indeed, an identity is an identity because its elements are recognizable over a given period of time. It is recognizable by certain characteristics or patterns, and these are what one group of people will to one degree or another point to (not always in a systematic or consistent manner) as defining what they consider to be factors marking them off from other groups of people. These characteristics may or may not coincide with some of what outsiders regard as distinctive about a group, as many theorists have pointed out.

However, precisely because of the vagueness of declared aspects of these identities, Barth's celebrated suggestion to fellow anthropologists is apposite to the understanding of ethnicity being advanced here (Barth 1969). He suggested that we should focus not so much on the elements of an ethnic identity, but pay attention to the boundaries that mark off one ethnicity from another. It is at these boundaries that differences are highlighted, thrown into sharp relief and at which points competition and conflict between groups may arise. The stress on the notion of 'the other' in many cultural studies of ethnicity may be located at these Barthian boundaries. It is also important, however, to say that the existence of such boundaries should be flexibly understood as boundaries where a great deal of fluidity exists. Expressed another way, it may be said that when sharp cultural differences exist side by side the boundaries necessarily become increasingly grey and vague. But at the same time as a group become sharply aware of their similarities and their differences, they also begin through a process of osmosis, so to speak, to borrow and lend characteristics across their borders or lines of demarcation.

This is what Malinowski (1961) described as 'culture contact' resulting in 'culture change'. The general point, however, is that no matter how we account for it, groups of people develop and identify shared characteristics, which also mark them off from other groups. And while these characteristics are susceptible to change, their endurance and transmission over space and time may be more significant in terms of how humans see themselves as social beings. The point here is not to set cultural susceptibility and imperviousness as absolutes, but perhaps more as points on a spectrum, depending on the situations or circumstances in which they find themselves.

It is important at this juncture to establish that the concept of ethnicity is conceptually and empirically distinct from that of 'race', although in practice these concepts are usually confused, collapsed together or overlapped in both academic and popular discourses. An example of this problem is the identity question posed by the British Office of National Statistics in the census of population in 1991 and 2001: here ethnic and racial as well as national identities are collapsed together (Goulbourne 2001). However, as a number of scholars have shown, these forms of identity are conceptually distinguishable (Cornell and Hartmann 1998). But this distinction between race and ethnicity is not as simple as it may appear. For example, it is possible – as in the UK – for people of different racial groups to share important aspects of ethnicity, while groups of people who are generally regarded to be very different may share the same racial identity, but not the same ethnic identity. Thus, African Caribbeans and indigenous Britons through the trajectories of history share significant aspects of ethnic identity – religion, language, customs, traditions. On the other hand, South Asians share with the indigenous population what anthropologists would regard as much the same racial heritage, but they may not share the same ethnic baggage – particularly with respect to the religious dimension of ethnicity.

The confusion of 'racial' and 'ethnic' identities also hides what Banton (2006) suggests is a relationship between 'folk' and analytical understandings and usages of a concept: in popular discourses the notions of 'racial' and 'ethnic' identities are interchanged, conflated and collapsed together. Consequently, there is an absence of analytical clarity or integrity to these concepts; the problem is compounded by an importation of concepts or notions from popular discourses into the analytical vocabulary. Any discussion on the street, in a pub or a restaurant or in an academic setting will confirm this kind of confusion of the popular and the analytical, each feeding on the other, and thereby providing a living for those academics, journalists and others who thrive on conceptual confusion. Of course, in the end, this may be of no consequence, particularly in a world of relativistic values, where one person's views are presumed to be as valid as those of the next person's – irrespective of the time and effort invested in the process of coming to their respective conclusions.

But clarity over these matters is not only about academic and intellectual integrity. At the level of social action – as distinguished from an exclusively conceptual understanding – these factors are reflected in several areas of British national life. For example, this is so in the effort to maintain newly invented ethnicities in

Britain – 'Asian', 'Caribbean' and others. Thus, while at a political or ideological level Asian and black people will unite to oppose racism and exclusion, there has hitherto been little social integration between these groups as expressed through marriage, conjugal partnerships, or other living arrangements; on the other hand, this is not uncommon between the indigenous or historic White population and both black and Asian minorities. Of course, as these different groups mix and mingle in the democratic context of post-imperial Britain, this situation is likely to change – despite the prescriptions of conservative multiculturalists (see, for example, Swann 1985; Parekh 2000), who go beyond the celebration and respect of difference to imply that it is a public good to maintain and develop present ethnic differences.

This perspective of ethnic and racial identities places an emphasis on discussion that is different from that which seeks to suggest there are no such differences between humans, and that the only real social phenomenon to be confronted is racism. To be sure, racism exists (see, for example, Back and Solomos, 2000) and is persistent – and we might call this popular or vulgar prejudicial racism. This is where a person's or a group's worth, beliefs and social action are taken to be determined by their racial identity. But there is also what we might call philosophical racism: this is where there is the belief that the physical differences between people are so fundamental that such differences override all social variables. In this view, as Banton pointed out some years ago, it is possible for a racist not to be negatively prejudicial at all, and might very well regard a person of another 'race' to be their equal (Banton 1967). Indeed, one example is the following formulation that is not uncommon, particularly in the USA, before and since the debate over race and intelligence reopened by the Bell Curve authors (Herrnstein and Murray 1994; Fraser 1995; Jacoby and Glaubermann 1995): East Asians (Chinese/Japanese) are intellectually superior to whites/Europeans; Europeans are superior to Africans/blacks; Africans/blacks are superior to others but only in athletics, and are intellectually inferior to others, and so on.

In this book we recognize that there are groups of people who wish to distinguish themselves from other groups of people by what they consider to be their 'racial' characteristics. This does not make them racists. Similarly, some groups may distinguish themselves from others by what they consider to be their 'ethnic identity', without being prejudicial in their relations with other ethnic groups. Such auto-description of communities to which individuals feel they belong will feature in the discussions that follow in Part II of this book. For now, concerns about families, community, and identities take us to the site of debates about social capital.

Social capital

It is generally assumed that families and communities – particularly communities demarcated by ethnic and/or racial identities – are sites rich in social capital that can be mined. The vast and growing literature on social capital – its meaning, access and use, its measurement, etc. – has been fairly exhaustively explored, particularly in the USA (see, for example, Putnam 2000; Arneil 2006). The concept is sometimes explicitly and sometimes implicitly employed to account for the fates of particular groups of new immigrants and others in the USA (see, for example, Foner 2001; Portes and Zhou 2001). If it was a little slow in crossing the Atlantic to Britain, for much of the first decade of the new century social capital arrived with some force hitting academic, policy/political and popular discourses at the same time (see, for example, Baron *et al.* 2000; Ruston 2001; Field 2003). In any event, the discussions about newcomers to post-Second World War Britain have long raised the same questions in Britain as are today discussed about social capital and new settler groups (see, Goulbourne 2008). What is necessary at this point, however, is an understanding of the concept of social capital to help us on our way better to grasp what may be happening to transnational families with bases in Britain.

We suggest that a working definition involves understanding social capital as a largely intangible and unquantifiable series of resources such as informal networks, and connections that are essentially social in the sense that the realization of its use-value is observable only where the individual or the group taps into it to produce or attain desired or beneficial results. Understood in this way, it may be taken that social capital is highly instrumental, pliable, even vague and slippery to pin down, and is not always observable. Indeed, it may be said that social capital is largely recognizable by its effect. Unlike material capital (land, minerals, money), social capital is largely invisible, and it is doubtful whether it can be taken to the formal or physical marketplace to be exchanged for other commodities; it is not likely to be taken to the stock market. It is largely, if not entirely, metaphor. However, this does not mean that social capital is entirely ethereal or epiphenomenal; it is real enough and its effects, if not its step-by-step procedures, observable and some scholars, researchers and policymakers believe that it can be calculated and is therefore measurable.

It may be obvious by now that we are more persuaded by Pierre Bourdieu (1997), Bourdieu and Passeron (1990) and their followers (see, for example, Arneil 2006), than we are by Robert Putnam and his disciples in discussions about social capital. This is because, while Bourdieu conveys a loose understanding of social capital and he grasps the fact that factors of social class, dominance and conflict are involved, Putnam's message tends to be far too certain and prescriptive. It goes without saying that Putnam's work on social capital has received a great deal of academic attention, and perhaps even more attention from policymakers/implementers and politicians in the polities across the Atlantic world. His message about the value of social capital in maintaining good communities has been received with reverence by governments, some civic organizations and others. In academic circles, Putnam's *Bowling Alone: The Collapse and Revival of American Community* (2000) has even been likened to Alexis de Tocqueville's *Democracy in America* (first published in 1835) and to other outstanding names and titles in the last century, such as C. Wright Mills and his work on the power elite in America. The message and its reception have bowled over many who are engaged with much the same set of issues as Putnam is concerned about, that is, the non-material or intangible values and resources (trust, bonding, support) that inform individual and community social action through such discreet networks as families and kinship units and a variety of community and other civic groups. In brief, Putnam's message is that contemporary American society no longer displays the sense of community that it did during what historians describe as the Progressive Age – the first decades of the twentieth century; that the sense of community held by Americans in the past was not only desirable in itself but is so for today's America.

Obviously, this all too skeletal representation does not convey the density and richness of Putnam's argument as any reader of his voluminous work and listener to his many presentations on both sides of the Atlantic will recognize. In addition, Putnam has gone on to argue that social capital is more likely to be in evidence in a homogeneous than a heterogeneous America (Putnam 2007); individuals in singular communities are more likely to be trusting than they are in pluralist communities. The apparent prescription from this observation might seem to be that society should strive to be singular, monocultural or homogeneous. The problem with this is that most human societies are heterogeneous, and within the context of globalization, as we will argue in the next chapter, the attainment of a singular, homogeneous and or monocultural society is likely to be the exception, not the rule. In any event, *dis-trust* is not always a negative. While trust is an obvious good, its opposite is not always necessarily dis-trust; this is because dis-trust is an essential feature of a questioning and therefore healthy democratic society (see, for example, Hart 1978; Goulbourne 2006).

One of the most powerful assaults on Putnam's work is Barbara Arneil's *Diverse Communities*, which is an incisive, thorough and honest critique of Putnam's much acclaimed work on social capital (Arneil 2006). Her work addresses the concept, diagnosis and prescription of social capital as articulated by Putnam, no doubt because he is the pre-eminent apostle or proponent of the *social-capitalogic* persuasion and who has caught the attention of the men and women – to paraphrase C. Wright Mills – whose wills prevail in the Atlantic world.

Arneil's central challenge of Putnam's thesis is this: while his work is meticulously documented (an undeniable fact), Putnam does not recognize that his golden age (the Progressive Era) in America when social capital was strong in civil society was also a time when for women, black Americans, and others this was a period of exclusion. The progressivism of the age was restricted to white men – and, as she might have added, only some white men. What has happened during the contemporary age, that Putnam bemoans, is the radical inclusion or participation of women and what Arneil, unfortunately, collapses into a rather meaningless category called 'cultural minorities' in American life – black Americans, communities of choice such as gays and lesbians and others. The wealth, so to speak, of social capital was not equitably distributed or available to all, and therefore the Progressive Age was not the paradise Putnam imagined. Arneil's several other points seem to flow from this major failure in Putnam's work. For example, the experiences or narratives of the dominated or excluded – groups of women, gay and lesbians, the disabled, Hispanics and African Americans – lay outside Putnam's account. Consequently, for Arneil, the assertion and recognition of issues about diversity and social justice on a broad front in contemporary America fail to accord with

Putnam's vision of what we may generally regard as the 'good' society. Arneil's central criticism is reinforced by a range of sophisticated arguments drawing on the women's movement, philanthropy and civil action, as well as political theory and the broader and critical perspectives of Pierre Bourdieu and other scholars who have focused on issues of democracy and trust – for example, Hart (1978) and Jean Cohen (1999).

Our understanding of social capital that is emerging in this discussion is informed by a critical if not an entirely sceptical perspective that calls for some explanation. First, while we view social capital as a useful heuristic device enabling us better to understand how some groups of people are able successfully to attain their desired ends, it is mostly when this social capital is used successfully that it is recognized. Groups that are judged to be successful are therefore deemed to have social capital; unsuccessful groups are equally assumed to be lacking in social capital. Part of Marx's critique of hoarding capital (the Spanish gold hording in the seventeenth century), was that potentially useful capital was not in circulation and therefore became rather useless; there needed to be commodities for gold as a currency to circulate in the market. It could also be the case that a group (a family, a kinship network, an ethnic community, etc.) may be rich in social capital, but because the group does not mobilize or use this capital it remains latent and therefore, as social capital, it is practically non-existent.

This dormancy aside, social capital identification appears largely to be a functional exercise; an understanding of social capital in this sense can therefore be rendered an exercise in tautology. What makes one group successful and another unsuccessful may very well not be the presence or absence of social capital but extraneous factors such as the possession of material wealth, political power and military force or wider, less tangible, factors such as cultural capital as explained by Coleman (see, Coleman 1988, 1990; Arniel 2006). With regard to racial and ethnic minorities in Britain, the experience of differential racism may be more responsible for differential outcomes or rewards than the nature or amount of social capital that they may be said to possess. If this line of reasoning has merit, then we need to be more critical about the utility of social capital.

Second, partly arising from this situation and partly independently, the question has to be asked whether it is not the case that one group's social capital may not be dysfunctionality for another group, depending on, for example, the socio-historical or psychological mixes of particular groups and communities, as well as specific circumstances or situations. For instance, the very fact of cultural proximity of Caribbeans to the majority culture of the historic UK population can be seen as being sometimes a social capital resource and at other times this proximity is a disadvantage. Similarly, the distance of most South Asian cultures from this same historically established majority culture is sometimes perceived as a distinct advantage in the development of Asian communities. While social capital denotes resources, it may nonetheless be a major mistake to see social capital as an unproblematic given – a given that necessarily can be identified and measured across different social groups and across 'ethnic', 'racial' and 'cultural' communities.

The concept of social capital shares a vagueness with the concept of ethnicity, and each leaves a kind of intellectual muddiness or cloudiness that inhibits comprehension of the social issues with which social capitologists and other social analysts want to grapple. Both concepts share the characteristics of being essentially social, as opposed to being individual and autonomous, and are not always easily pinned down. In character they are both chameleon-like, changing colours according to the circumstances or situations being confronted.

As indicated earlier, social capital, as the term suggests, is usually distinguished from human and economic capital: the former (education, training, skills) informs the latter (financial, land, minerals, etc.) by preparing the individual to compete in an ostensibly free marketplace. The individual – that being who is to be found everywhere in classical liberal political economy, politics and sociology – possesses these forms of capital. Whether we consider Marx's 'free' worker whose labour-power is alienated, Durkheim's disconnected or anomic individual or Weber's staunch Protestant/Calvinist individual, the relationship between people and the wider world is individualized within post-Reformation, capitalist or modern society. This individual is travelling much farther and much faster in current postmodernist social thinking, but remains crucial to the understanding of modern societies, including the different forms of capital.

The growing body of literature on social capital agrees that this is a form of capital that is collectively possessed and utilized – hence its elusiveness. Its collective quality suggests that social capital is not a commodity that can, like little piggy, be taken to market in exchange for another independent commodity. In other words, social capital is not actually a commodity exchangeable through other forms of free-floating commodities; it may have little meaning or use outside the social group. While other forms of capital – land, minerals, money – may have their own limitations, they may be less dependent on the social group to be activated. Marx's labourer or proletariat possesses one thing that can be commoditized – labour power, time – and this is quantifiable and therefore marketable. The general attractiveness of the concept of social capital would appear partly to be that it is a kind of catch-all or residual category of resource which cannot convincingly be fitted into the categories of material capital (land, water, buildings, minerals, money, etc.). It appears to allow us to bring into closer focus differential possession of resources that affects outcomes in a competitive society. It is easy enough therefore to dismiss the concept as being too vague, but there is also a duty to exercise care in order not to slip into mystification on the one hand, and on the other, not to be so sceptical as entirely to dismiss the concept out of hand.

Following Baron, *et al.*'s (2000) suggestion, we utilized the concept of social capital as a heuristic device to help us better to understand the complex relationships between the family, ethnicity and community dynamics of our work. We found the notions of 'bonding', 'bridging' and 'linking' social capital highly suggestive, but, as with the more general concept of social capital, their utility lies in the power of metaphor. This power is that of teasing out potentially useful lines of questioning, following through lines of enquiry and discussion about possibilities. These do not always end in conclusive observations, but they do help to interrogate raw data in order to find meanings about the lives of families and communities. Bonding social capital is just what the word 'bonding' suggests: building and maintaining trust between individuals who believe that they share certain things, such as beliefs and values; they can rely on each other, and this may involve such emotional factors as love, affection, common likes and dislikes and so forth. Bonding suggests that individuals do not always have to return to first principles in order to explain or justify choices and preferences in social action. Bonding cements an individual's effective membership of a family or a kinship group, of civic associations and of broader institutions such as a political party or a faith group. Bonded groups of people are necessarily demarcated from other similarly bonded groups, but they may be 'linked' or certain factors may act as a 'bridge'; these two kinds of social capital strongly emphasize the metaphoric value of the concept.

In Britain, until the last decade or so, the concept of social capital was not generally or widely utilized in academic discussion about ethnicity, although some specific public policy initiatives invited consideration of such relationships. However, important aspects of the concerns of social capital theorists have been more than strongly implied in several debates about ethnicity, and race and ethnic relations in Britain over the past three or four decades. A key assumption that informs much of the work in migrant communities and race relations analyses has been that some groups are better equipped than others to draw upon family, kinship and communal resources.

For example, it has been asserted that the different kinds of participation of minority ethnic groups in Britain have been determined by the value systems of these groups – perhaps the central concept in the vocabulary of theorists who may be described as social capitalogists. According to this view, there are two strong models of participation of minority ethnic communities in British society: the Jewish (represented as being socially, economically and politically successful, and well integrated into the upper echelons of society) and the Irish (generally represented as being less successful and mainly outside the mainstream of British society). Subsequent groups, the argument goes on, followed this dual pattern. Thus, while Asians are assumed to have followed the Jewish model of incorporation, African Caribbeans are assumed to have followed the example of the Irish. To one degree or another these views were widely expressed in the 1970s and 1980s with regard to the economy (see, for example, Ward and Jenkins 1984), and political participation (Rex and Tomlinson 1979; Dench 1986; Jacob 1986). Indeed, the view that Caribbeans withdraw from political engagement has been reflected in a recent assessment (McLean, 2002) of their participation in community organizations, and this is now seen (mistakenly) as a comment on these group's stock of social capital.

In the main, what used to be described as the value systems of respective minority ethnic groups are not very dissimilar to what are now referred to as social capital. While the social capital debate may more clearly focus attention on aspects of cultural values and behaviour than did earlier debates about values, it should be noted that the emphasis which some scholars placed on the role of racism (see, Solomos 1991; Back and Solomos 2000) as an inhibiting factor in the differential outcomes of groups, is set aside by the social capitalogists: the performance or form of integration of groups appears to depend entirely on what cultural baggage they arrived with at their destination.

This neglect of the role of racism is strongly reflected in the literature on minority ethnic communities in America, where interest in families and social capital has been more manifest than in Britain. In both countries researchers have been overwhelmingly concerned about questions of integration or the forms of incorporation of immigrants and their offspring into the majority society. In the USA, however, the scale of immigration from a wider range of societies than Britain, has stimulated and maintained a long tradition of interest in how newcomers, distinguished by race and ethnicity, integrate into the social order. The origins of this tradition or interest is often attributed to Chicago School sociologists of the 1920s and 1930s, particularly the work of Park (1950). But, arguably, W. E. B. Du Bois' (1973) work in Philadelphia in the last years of the nineteenth century and followed by his sketches and essays *The Souls of Black Folks* (1903) has a greater claim to this status (see, Lewis 1993). The maintenance of separate communities alongside each other in the USA, each of which participates in the market and together united by the forces of production of goods and their exchange, has been based on an overall commodity-plenty society, including abundance of space in relation to population. In a space-limited, historically honed population, relatively homogenous culture and highly centralized nation-state, such as post-imperial Britain into which new immigrant communities have been inserted or incorporated, the question of integration has become equally or more pressing, and this is reflected in both the academic and policy worlds. In this situation there are at least three important observations to bear in mind from the longer and more developed American concern with integration.

First, this body of literature places a strong emphasis on comparison between ostensibly different groups, as well as their perceived and experiential differential incorporation into American society. In this literature we are invited to look at the differential performance of communities in terms of success and failure, assessed by degrees of acquisition of wealth, occupation, residence and general life chances. These groups or communities come from a variety of societies in the Old World (Europe, Asia, Africa) and from within the New World (the Caribbean, Central America, South America). It is not irrelevant to say that this practice of comparing stands in a respectable Aristotelian tradition of endowing validity to evidence selected or brought together through a process of assessing similarity and dissimilarity of human experiences and the institutions which arise from such experiences and reasoning.

There is, however, a limitation to how this methodology is sometimes utilized in both societies: by freezing a given moment and ignoring the past, there is a tendency to belittle or undermine the changes that occur within and between groups, as well as within families and kinship groups, as a result of culture contact. There is a general tendency to take the present moment as representative of total reality. This is persuasive for at least two reasons: first, concentrating on the moment conveys a strong sense of scientific method and therefore of validity or truth; the fact also that experience and perceptions are conveyed through the agency of objective numbers (supported by graphs and tables) make this method particularly attractive to different publics: politicians, administrators, journalists and so forth. The powerful corrections provided by history or the longer view of human experience, our uncertainty about the future, and the range and variety of human creativity (not all morally acceptable to all) are wittingly or unwittingly set aside as irrelevant to the sociological account of lived experience.

We must, nonetheless, understand the attraction and basis of comparison. We can identify some of these as being the benevolent drive towards equality for all in a multicultural society, active participation within communities, and social cohesion as expressed by so many state policy initiatives, particularly since the mid-1990s in Britain. For example, the Social Exclusion Unit and the Policy Action Teams in the Cabinet Office have recognized that 'minority ethnic communities are at disproportionate risk of social exclusion' (Cabinet Office 2000: 7), and drawing on the many reports about the nature of their disadvantages in housing and neighbourhood renewal, education and training, employment, health and so forth, have stressed the need to incorporate their needs and the issues which arise into overall government policies. While the government does not have something called a social capital strategy, it is nonetheless the case that notions that are derived from social capital thinking inform discussions about neighbourhood renewal, family, community, citizenship and so forth. These are all conceived in terms of collective social action, and it may be argued that particularly within the context of a multicultural society the notion of social capital is attractive.

Of course, the ideal of the multicultural society as put forward by some of its most strident advocates (see for example, Rex and Tomlinson 1979; Swann 1985; Parekh 2000) may promote toleration and require social peace, but it may also conflict with the notion of a cohesive society. The Home Office (Ruston 2001) places great emphasis on promoting what they describe as 'active' communities, race equality and the family. But these relate to the notion of social capital and in general draw upon Putnam's (2000) and particularly Woolcock's work (1998), emphasizing social networks, reciprocity and trust and anchored around his break-down of social capital as 'bridging' (between different groups/communities; outward-looking), 'bonding' (inward-looking, reinforcing bonds within groups), and 'linking' (linking local networks across the country). Each of these resonates with past normative accounts of group behaviour, from the group theorists at the beginning of the twentieth century in France, Britain and the USA (see, for example, Nicholls 1974; Bentley 1908), to discussions in past decades about inward-looking and outward-looking ethnic communities, or indeed to discussions in politics about different kinds of community political engagement and participation since the 1970s (see, for example, Dahl 1961; Milbrath 1965; Birch 1993).

Second, the American tradition of enquiry into racial and ethnic identity and solidarity as applied to the field of family studies, sets out questions which may be quantified or measured by widely acceptable empirical criteria. Thus, there are questions about a wide range of issues to do with ethnicity, family and social capital, such as education, employment and residence (see, for example, Bianchi and Robinson 1997; Driessen 2001). The same degree of attention has not been evident in Britain, but this may be forthcoming since the need for at least a modicum of social cohesion in a post-imperial multicultural society is becoming increasingly evident (Goulbourne 1991; Ouseley 2001).

A number of issues remain to be addressed fully in empirical research: for example, the extent to which ethnicity is perceived, utilized and reproduced as social capital or resource in the processes of lived family life; what it might mean to say that ethnic values and solidarity affect or condition family behaviour and structure/ organization, particularly in conditions where communities are adjusting to new situations such as in multicultural Britain where different cultures meet; and how ethnicity – understood as social capital – is reproduced within the discrete domains of families and kinship relationships across national boundaries. We need to ask questions about the conditions necessary for ethnic affinities to become a family resource or a social commodity; whether families are the most effective conduit for maintaining ethnic social bonding across national state boundaries; and, crucially, whether groups that appear to lack ethnic solidarity are refusing to mobilize their ethnicity or capitalize their shared ethnic values. In the British context, this kind of research should help us to explore such questions as whether the high level of inter-ethnic marriage/partnership threatens or strengthens ethnic solidarity or opens the way to a new and more tolerant and inclusive national culture. In addition, it should also allow us some insight into whether the possession and utilization of multiple ethnic and nation-state identities are likely to be the future direction of a regional (of continental proportion) if not a global social order.

Conclusion: a tripartite or a quadripartite relationship?

In the substantive discussion in this chapter we have argued that we have moved from a trinity of three concepts or constructs of families, ethno-racial identities and communities to the fourth notion of social capital. The relationship is not, therefore, a holistic trinity, but one that is quite elastic and can expand to include other conceptual constructions. Several of the problems and issues discussed in this chapter are addressed empirically in Part II of this book, but before moving on to these it is necessary to continue the general exploration of some key concerns. The next chapter, therefore, outlines some questions about how we framed our research questions, collected our data and sought to gain understanding from them about social life.

3 Methodological issues and challenges

Introduction

We have so far seen what are some of the drawbacks and strengths of current thinking about transnational families, social capital, communities and related issues arising from these agencies and forces in modern societies. In this chapter, we move on to consider some of the methodological challenges posed by our comparative and collaborative project in understanding the changing forms of transnational families in societies such as that of Britain. This is because one of our main aims is to use particular family experiences to go beyond or transcend descriptions and understandings of families who cross national boundaries. We consider whether there are meaningful commonalities across experiences otherwise separated by identities of every kind – racial and ethnic, gender and sexual, generational and so forth. An account of the methodology we employed in collecting data for our analysis is therefore placed at this point in our discussion.

Research questions and relevance

We start with the broad research questions to which we wanted some answers about transnational families and communities in Britain. As noted in Chapter 1, understanding transnational families is not merely a matter of examining families in different locations communicating with each other across national boundaries. To be sure, transnational families do communicate across national boundaries; they also communicate across other boundaries such as those defined by ethnicities, cultures, racial identities, nationality and so forth. But, as stated in Chapter 1, we want to go beyond this 'taken for granted' understanding of the transnational nature or dimension of family lives and identify some elements that may be common across the political boundaries of the nation-state, and the identities of 'race' and ethnicity, gender, generation and so forth.

Of course, all research projects start with a set of questions or hypotheses about social action, structures and perceptions, whether these are explicit or implicit. These questions or hypotheses are general assumptions or assertions about our subject that guide us in the activity of collecting new data or reinterpreting existing knowledge about social life. Research questions also help to guide the researcher in selecting relevant problems, issues and patterns as well as highlight absences in the assembled data. We therefore commenced our empirical research into transnational families by asking the following pertinent questions:

- Are there some necessary conditions for ethnic affinities to become a family resource or a social commodity?
- Do families become the conduit for transforming ethnic affinities in a multi-ethnic/plural society and across national state boundaries?
- Are groups that appear to lack ethnic solidarity refusing to mobilize their ethnicity or capitalize shared ethnic values?
- Does inter-ethnic marriage/partnership threaten or strengthen ethnic solidarity in a multicultural Britain, or does it open new challenges and possibilities?
- Are families a significant site for actively undermining national identity based on race and ethnicity and therefore changing the overall social order?
- What are the implications of the possession and utilization of multiple ethnic and nation-state identities?

Our general perspective that transnational families involve the lived experiences of family members scattered across national boundaries fractures or compromises the nationalist ideal that all members of a particular nation-state share a common heritage and destiny, or that the nation-state divide is necessarily the most important or significant in the lives of individuals who live and have their existence on a given territory or a country. In a previous chapter we also saw how the communities that people as collectives or and individuals form are not necessarily restricted to space or indeed time, but may and do cross these boundaries not only in their memories and aspirations but also in their daily lived experiences. In order to capture and understand these experiences, it was necessary to initiate and develop an appropriate methodology that was comparative and transnational in character.

First, as noted in Chapter 1, our collaborative work involved bringing together individual scholars from different academic disciplines who had different but shared or overlapping intellectual concerns and who came to the enterprise with different generational experiences. The reports or dissemination of most research projects – particularly products from the research, such as articles and books – rarely outline this aspect of the total research process. This aspect is more often than not a silent dimension. To be sure, there are exceptions, and two examples are in order. Particularly in family studies, what may spring readily to the minds of some readers is the insistence in feminist methodology that there should be a degree of reflection on the research methodology or process by researchers during the writing up stage of these matters (De Vault 1996; Chafetz 1997; Maynard and Purvis 1994; Hemmings 2005; Laslett 2007). Thus, some researchers have indeed pointed to the strengths, weaknesses and the opportunities provided in the field and the need to be adaptable to changing situations (see, Cowan and Goulbourne 2001; Edwards 2004).

In the broader social science community there is the insistence in historical social studies that sound research must take account of the problem or tension in the relationship between the object and the subject in the study of human society and social action. Nowhere, perhaps, are these concerns more clearly stated than in the works of Max Weber and Gunnar Myrdal, and for this reason it is worth briefly considering the relevance of their thoughts for our enterprise.

Weber insisted that we set aside what he called 'our demonic position' (our particular prejudices, values, etc.) from the task of analysing and accounting for social action in human societies (Lassman and Velody 1988; Swedberg 2003). While not the unabashed positivist that Émile Durkheim and some of his disciples were (for example, Talcott Parsons) Weber nonetheless thought that social processes and action could be relatively objectively described so that the subjectivity of the researcher or writer does not override the 'truth' or 'fair' understanding of a given social situation, or what Durkheim might have called 'representations' of social aspects of our lives. Thus, for Weber, social studies or the study of human society and action was an interpretive act or decision, or an undertaking of interpreting the meanings of what we as humans do or do not do.

For Gunnar Myrdal, writing later in the 1940s, there was an equal or even stronger insistence that we distinguish the researcher's subjective 'valuations' or value-judgements from the object of analysis or the situation being studied. Perhaps Myrdal sets out his case more systematically in his *Objectivity in Social Research* (1970), but when his arguments are read as part of his influential *An American Dilemma: The Negro Problem and Modern Democracy* (1944), published in the midst of the war against German fascism and Japanese expansionism, the admonition takes on added force. Like Weber, Myrdal was an economist but, when analysing and describing social life and action, both men sought to pinpoint the moral philosopher's distinction between 'ought' and 'is' questions.

For both scholars, the social analyst is always on the horn of the dilemma of choosing between their preferences and the reality of what exists. Since we cannot fully arrive at or describe the 'real' (of a situation, or an event), then for Weber we must recognize that as a human person the social analyst must be prepared to be content to 'interpret the meaning of social action and thereby give a causal explanation of the way in which the action proceeds and the effects which it produces' (Weber 1995: 70). For Myrdal it was crucial that as a social analyst the researcher recognizes that he 'is part of the culture in which he lives, and he never succeeds in freeing himself entirely from dependence on the dominant preconceptions and biases of his environment' (Myrdal 1944: 1035).

For both Myrdal and Weber the researcher of social life is 'more or less entangled ... in the web of conflicting valuations' (ibid.), and, as Myrdal stressed about black America (the subject of his research), 'even the scientific biases will run against the Negroes most of the time' (ibid.), thereby strongly questioning the nature or degree of the attainment of the objectivity of social analysis. This was a point emphasized by Frantz Fanon (1968, 1970) who argued that bias in scientific enquiry about human situations is nearly always directed against the colonized, not the colonizer – a point that goes back to the mantra of historians that in general history is written from the perspective of the victor, not the defeated, from the perspective of the dominant, not the subordinated. In short, the researcher's 'value-judgements' (Weber) or 'valuations' (Myrdal) are based on our ethical standards, ideals, our worldviews. We need not, however, entirely agree with Weber in insisting that the tensions involved here are 'irresolvable' because 'the question cannot be discussed in scientific terms, since it is itself entirely dependent on practical value-judgements' (Weber 1995: 69), unless we understand resolution for this problem to be absolutely possible.

Neither of these major contributors to the study of society entirely resolved the problem of the relationship between subject and object, between subjectivity and objectivity. Indeed, the wisdom they imparted suggested that this will always be a point of contention, with which we live. However, since the analysis of social life and action has a practical aspect – namely, our understandings of social phenomena informing our social action – then we have to content ourselves with the best that we can do and muddle-through, so to speak. In this regard, neither man entirely abandoned the enterprise of attaining statements about social life and action that could be generally accepted about our human situation or social action. They suggested that we delimit the permeation of biases by first making explicit our own values or standpoints, developing hypotheses, and drawing practical conclusions from our research findings. This suggestion placed an emphasis on 'relevance': the relevance of selection, or what Myrdal called 'the principle of selection' about 'the practical aspects of social problems' (Myrdal 1944: 1060).

In recent decades researchers have been more modest, or less ambitious, than were our predecessors in the late nineteenth century and the first half of the twentieth century about the power of science and the presumed scientific method to help us understand and explain social life. Perhaps for Myrdal more than for Weber, social studies are a political science because of their practical outcomes or implications. We will return to this point of the relevance of research for the practical world in which families live in a transnational world in the concluding chapter of this book. In the rest of this chapter it is relevant briefly to consider some of the practical experiences of conducting research into transnational families based in Britain with functional links in different parts of the world.

The interview, life-story narration and social analysis

Given that our overall aim was to understand the emerging patterns of British families with recent and continuing links across the globe, we were faced with the practical problem of selection. That is to say, how do we choose which families to include and which to exclude from our study. Combining Myrdal's 'principle of selection' and his emphasis on good research being based on 'relevance' to practical issues and problems in society, we chose to focus on British families with continuing links in three regions of the world which have significantly fashioned the making of post-imperial British society. These are the Commonwealth Caribbean, the Indian sub-continent, and southern Europe. As will be explained in the next chapter, there are people from other parts of the world who have had significant impacts on contemporary British society, particularly London metropolitan life. However, it was not practical to include representations of all these communities, and it was not necessary to do so in order to find answers to our research questions.

We collected qualitative data through in-depth, one-to-one interviews across the national boundaries of Britain, three Commonwealth Caribbean countries (Barbados, Jamaica and Guyana), two Indian states (Goa and Punjab),[1] and two regions in Italy (Trentino and Sicily). In Britain we identified areas of sizeable settlement by people from these countries and regions, and interviews of individuals were conducted across generations of individual family members with heritages linking these sites in different countries.

For the Commonwealth Caribbean we interviewed 100 individuals (54 men and 46 women) between 16 and 30 years of age with backgrounds in Barbados, Guyana and Jamaica. The emphasis in this project was to examine how British young people derive their understandings of identities across national boundaries. In Britain, the interviews were conducted in London, Birmingham, Manchester and Nottingham, because we wanted to concentrate on areas of intense Caribbean settlement as well as some less research-frequented areas of settlement. Areas of sizeable return-settlements in our three Caribbean countries were also visited and interviews conducted. In Barbados we conducted interviews in the parishes (the administrative divisions of the country) of Bridgetown (also the country's capital), St James, and St Michael. Interviews in Guyana were held in the capital city of Georgetown, and the regions of Berbice and East and West Demerara. In Jamaica interviews were carried out in the capital city of Kingston and parishes in different parts of the country – St Andrew, St Ann, St James, St Mary, Manchester and Portland.

The second project on transnational families and social capital on which we draw in this book explored some important rituals about the inner workings of families, households and communities in British families of Italian backgrounds, and focused on the mutual provision of care as social capital. Participant observations, case studies, and 50 in-depth interviews were undertaken across three generations of British families of Italian backgrounds in Aylesbury, Bedford, London, Oxford and Peterborough. In the Italian homeland we also conducted 25 interviews of individuals of the same families.

Our main methodology was therefore essentially subjective. This was because we were concerned to address the subjective feelings, beliefs and perceptions of members of families and their communities as distinct from whatever the general and sometimes more objective understandings may be of these different families and communities. In order to attain the understanding we sought about these families, we conducted mainly one-to-one, face-to-face interviews of individual members of families living in Britain and the specific places mentioned earlier in the Caribbean, Italy and India. Interviews were tape-recorded and later transcribed, and of course, we observed the ethical convention of anonymizing the names of our respondents, and sometimes also specific local place names where these could be relatively easily recognized. Family studies are a sensitive area of social studies, and so the one-to-one approach is of vital importance in conducting such research. It allows the respondent to express their views about significant aspects of their individual lives, as well as the complexity of their relationships with their senses of identity, members of their immediate families, their wider kinship network, friends, and significant others outside the boundaries into which they were born and socialized. Individual self-reflections and comments about subjective experiences can be painful as well as therapeutic and enjoyable for respondents, but in the end the data collected in the interview exchange is deeply personal and demands the respect of the researcher in how these are recorded, analysed and portrayed in publications.

The subjective method, however, allows the researcher to capture much of the dynamism, contradictions, pleasures and the *angst* of personal biographies from the perspectives of specific persons who are also agents of social continuities and social change. The in-depth one-to-one interview has long provided social researchers with a major means of collecting data about discrete aspects of social, economic and political life. But more recently, historians who have long depended on such artefacts as written records, dates and events have rediscovered the oral tradition, and with this the profound importance of the voices of ordinary people in the construction of narratives of lived lives. In this regard, of particular relevance is the work of Paul Thompson. Building on Vansina's (1965) emphasis on the use of memory and the oral history tradition in preliterate societies, Thompson has constructed a body of work about the lives of ordinary people by gathering data through interviewing individuals about their lives (see, for example, Thompson 1978). The technique allows the individual to tell their story in their own words. These individuals are allowed as much time as they wish to express themselves. The interview questionnaire serves as a guide and not as a rigid control of the dialogue that ensues in a successful interview. Focused around specific aspects of the individual's life – education, occupation, the cycle of family life, community membership and activities and so forth – the method has proven to be very valuable to social historians and sociologists.

In social history investigation, Trevor Lummis, a student of Thompson's, is of particular importance because, while being conscious of the method's many challenges, Lummis demonstrated how the oral history method can be used to enhance our understanding of the past of non-writing, discrete communities. The title of Lummis' book *Listening to History* (1987) is itself suggestive of the strength of this method of constructing the past from the lived experiences of the living. In sociology an apt illustration of the oral history method is Ken Plummer's work. Plummer has been a member of the same sociology department as Thompson at the University of Essex, and it can be imagined that they may have influenced each other. Plummer (2003) sets forth what he calls a 'transformation schema', involving the telling of stories in five stages: imaging (visualizing, empathizing with a cause), articulating (vocalizing, announcing), inventing identities (becoming storytellers), creating social worlds (communities of support), creating a culture of public problems. He applied his schema to the origins, development, and tolerance of male homosexuality and lesbianism in society, but the model could be applied to a range of social phenomena in modern societies, and certainly to family studies.

Going further back to studies in politics and sociology, we find that the work of Eric Schattschnieder (1967) and Charles Wright Mills (1970) anticipated this perception of larger social problems. In the late 1950s, Mills suggested that we make a distinction between our individual problems and public issues, and emphasized how the one may be transformed into the other. Similarly, in the 1930s Schattschnieder had stressed how weaker parties in a conflict would try to make that conflict contagious so as to make the outcome less predictable, while the stronger party would want to contain the scope of the conflict so as to make the outcome favourable to themselves.

But, in the end, irrespective of how we plan and describe the method of how we gather data and analyse it, the researcher is still left with the heavy responsibility of interpreting the data collected. This is where we do not agree with those who hold that the data speaks for itself or that the care taken with the method or technique employed in collecting the data so tightly includes or incorporates the views or voices of respondents (whom they tend to call informants, as if research data is neutral). We insist that data collected by whatever means require selection, analysis and interpretation, and the process involved must weigh the views, testimonies and perceptions of respondents against other evidences or perceptions. As analysts, therefore, we take full responsibility for the views offered in this book. And while in our empirical analyses we incorporate the voices of respondents as much as is reasonable, we do not wish to suggest that the data from our respondents speak directly to the reader. We bear the responsibility of being interpreters or analysts of the data, and this behoves us briefly to describe aspects of the research process in the field.

The research process

It is neither possible nor necessary to tell the total story of the research process as a social problem or issue. This is because the process is complex, overlapping with a variety of other processes and the different intertwinings of persons, events, accidents, opportunities and setbacks are not all equally interesting. In any event, researchers are fundamentally more concerned to tell the story of their results or findings than they are to describe the various twists and turns from start to finish. It is always useful, however, to outline aspects of the adventure of research in the field, and in this section we want briefly to mention some of the factors we encountered. In particular, we want briefly to comment on the problems of selection and access, the insider/outsider status of the researcher, and ethical conduct.

First, research into families and communities is a delicate and sensitive matter and therefore selection and access require careful consideration and negotiation. We have explained elsewhere the broad basis of our selection of the communities in this study, but there were other levels and issues of selection, and of access. In the first instance, formal letters of introduction and a brief explanation of the aim and objectives of the project were sent to key persons and organizations to request a meeting to discuss our project and thereby begin the negotiation for access to potential interviewees. These initial face-to-face meetings with community representatives were usually formal and we would be questioned about the nature and purpose of the research. Indeed, on a number of occasions we had to explain the study before a committee and respond to their questions. We were also encouraged to answer questions about our own personal backgrounds such as: 'Where are you from?', 'What country or region are your parents from?' We also had to allay concerns that we would not negatively represent respondents' families and communities. Naturally, these negotiations were lengthy and time-consuming because we had to go through two, sometimes three, tiers of 'gatekeepers' within communities and organizations. At each tier, new 'gatekeeper' relationships would be cultivated so that trust could be established, and sometimes reaffirmed.

Once trust was established we were passed on to the next tier of 'gatekeeper', such as individuals working more directly within communities, people who could help us with potential interviewees. These meetings were much less formal and shorter in length because there was trust in the person who had referred us. In these instances, second-tier 'gatekeepers' often required only basic information about the project and reassurances about confidentiality and anonymity before they identified people to participate in the study. By this time, the interviewees with whom we spoke generally asked us few questions and were happy to participate in the study because we had already established trust relationships at previous stages.

There were other resources that we drew upon to access participants. For example, in the case of the Italian study our researcher participated in two conferences organized by a regional Italian government in Brussels, Belgium and Trentino, Italy, on youth of Italian origin. Although not directly on the topic of our research, these conferences provided us with invaluable information about Italian emigrants and communities across the world and enabled us to make initial contact with Italians living in London. Although we had already gone down the route of trying to contact participants through Italian Church groups and other organizations in London, attending these conferences and meeting some 'key' people, who acted as 'gatekeepers', speeded up and facilitated the process of access. At a very practical level, having specific persons' names and organizations we could mention in a phone call, helped our interlocutors to have a sense of who we were and facilitated the establishment of trust. We recognized that other Italian migrants and offspring often agreed to be interviewed as a favour to the people who had given us their names. In both the Italian project and those relating to India and the Caribbean we benefited from other persons' social capital.

But using our participants' networks was not always a successful shortcut to achieve our goals. Indeed, while the mapping of their transnational networks in the UK, other countries of destination, and their homelands in the Caribbean and Italy were central to our research, this approach raised some methodological questions. For example, during our interviews we became aware that our choice of one network over another – or our opportunity to gain access to one and not another network – would influence the outcome of the research. Early in our fieldwork we recognized the implications of following up the networks of specific individuals, because individuals and groups build relationships of trust, reciprocity and shared values, and as a result the circle of people contacted through one participant tended to have many characteristics in common. Our dilemma became whether to try to investigate some networks in depth, or to diversify and present as broad a picture as possible by taking into account a number of smaller networks. We decided that both options were valid for what we wanted to achieve.

Second, we found that the identity of the researcher was of significance in the field. Each researcher had an 'insider' knowledge of the communities being studied, and this status provided us with an understanding of the underlying rationale of the 'vetting' process in gaining access. In this we were able to utilize our own social capital to develop particular strategies to address the concerns of potential participants. We created project leaflets and distributed these at meetings with organizations and associations we approached for assistance. The leaflets included photographs of the research team members and brief details of the university; this helped to promote the notion of 'sameness' of researchers and researched. We also produced a 'frequently asked questions' leaflet that provided information about our role as the researcher, and addressed issues around analysis and reporting of the data.

For example, with respect to Caribbeans, we were aware that a shared racial and cultural positioning with the 'gatekeepers' would in itself not be enough to guarantee access, because Caribbean communities in Britain have a sophisticated understanding of the research process. We knew that our initial request to participate in the research might be treated with suspicion, because some researchers have pathologized and created misconceptions about Caribbean communities in Britain, and there is consequently what Goulbourne *et al.* (1995) described as 'research fatigue' in these communities. Although our use of 'gatekeepers' enabled us to access a diverse range of participants within a relatively short time, we also recognized a number of problems with this approach. We were mindful that the 'gatekeepers' might direct us towards participants who best represented the interests of organizations or their own interests, and that the access granted by the 'gatekeepers' revealed their own investments in maintaining and developing particular social networks, and also their own particular interests or bias. We were therefore aware that 'gatekeepers' exercised power in allowing or denying access to individual members and within community groups and associations, and they tended to speak for and on behalf of others who had junior and less powerful status.

There are some obvious advantages in working with one's own ethnic group. These can include a shared racial/ethnic consciousness, speaking the language (in case of migrants groups where English is not the first language), and being generally more aware of the cultural norms and practices of the people we study. In addition, we already knew many individuals in the respective ethnic groups we were researching, which speeded up the process. However, even in instances where we did not have prior knowledge, contacts or an understanding of local norms and values (as for example with our fieldwork in the multiple locations and regions of the Caribbean and Italy), because of a shared ethnic background, individuals were very willing to offer extra help in identifying others for interview. A shared ethnicity enabled us to build a rapport with our interviewees, who believed that we would be better equipped to understand their experiences.

Of course, a shared ethnicity also posed problems during the research process. We recognized that our participants were likely to feel under scrutiny from an interviewer whom they thought shared cultural values and who could judge their behaviour against specific norms. Indeed, it was very common for our potential interviewees to ask a number of personal questions in order to understand our positions on a range of issues, spanning across family life, politics, and religion. They felt sufficiently comfortable and confident with us to feel they could make moral judgements about our personal lives, even if we did not conform to expected cultural norms.

There were also other problems that resulted from a shared ethnic identity, some of which were of an ethical nature. It is widely recognized that people change their ethnic identification according to circumstances, and during the course of study we too became aware that we were constructing our ethnicity and deploying it strategically. In the Italian context, for example, we know that immigrants from Italy tend to have a weak sense of themselves as Italians *qua* Italians; rather, they tend more to identify with the locality they are from. Regional origins have great importance for both Italian emigrants and Italians in Italy, so that some commentators speak of the presence of regional ethnicities rather than of a national one (for example, Maffioletti 2004). Thus, one of our researchers, of Italian origin, started to draw on her own regional identity during the fieldwork. There were instances where we 'adjusted' our ethnic identity in accordance with the identity of our audience or interviewee. For examples in the Italian context, self-definitions varied from being Trentina (in the north) to being Sicilian (in the south). Similarly, in the Caribbean it was necessary to relate to the different identities of Barbadians, Guyanese and Jamaicans; not unlike Italians, Caribbeans have a far stronger sense of their island and territorial identities than of being Caribbeans or West Indians.

Importantly, we used this 'insider' status to negotiate our 'insider/outsider' positioning and utilized 'bonding' and 'bridging' social capital within these groups and networks. A range of social norms governed the negotiation process and our knowledge and ability to negotiate with these group norms and practices reflected both our 'insider' research positioning and 'bonding' social capital. A main benefit of being positioned as 'insider' is that it provided us with additional insight and knowledge of the community being studied. Our experience of the Caribbean community, for instance, led us to expect that, without personal connection, it would be difficult to access groups and individuals. From the onset, therefore, we anticipated that we would have to establish some shared ground, and work at cultivating and facilitating trust relationships.

Our 'insider' status and 'insider' knowledge of how social networks develop within the Caribbean and Italian communities meant that we had a 'taken for granted' understanding of sites such as black-led and Italian churches, and we considered community associations to be the best points to begin 'snowballing'. Even in instances where we did not have any contacts within community organizations, we utilized our social capital to approach existing contacts whom we knew could facilitate our access into these groups or played up our institutional position as academic researchers. This process in turn provided us with a wealth of social and cultural resources that we could further utilize.

Finally, in rounding up the discussion of our experience in the field, we must stress that our account so far suggests a number of complex ethical issues faced by researchers in the human sciences, particularly in the intimate regions of family and community studies. For example, in addition to contacting individuals through community organizations and regional associations, we used our personal, family and friendship networks to identify potential participants. In these instances access to individuals or groups were relatively straightforward because a 'trust-based relation' (Field 2003: 64) was already established, and we could use these (direct and indirect) personal connections for the collective benefit of this relatively large-scale collaborative research enterprise. However, using family and personal relationships in this way raises moral and ethical questions for the researcher that are rarely discussed. We were faced with questions such as whether, as researchers, we were exploiting intimate, familial trust-based relationships for personal gain or for the purpose of research. Another question we faced was that of the extent to which participants (accessed through friends or family) take part in the study because of a genuine interest in the research or because of a commitment to their friendships or imitate relationships. While this second question may not in the end matter too much – after all, there must be a variety of reasons why individuals choose to participate in social research – it did occur to us that the motive for such 'voluntary' participation warrants at least a modicum of reflection about the research process. Discussions about research relationships and the social and cultural resources drawn upon by researchers, as well as the moral and ethnical issues experienced in the research process, could be more forcefully integrated into parts of social analysis.

This point may be clearly illustrated by one example from our Italian research experience. When we contacted the leader of an Italian regional association, he kindly invited us to his organization's management meeting and explained to members who we were and what we were doing. Having met us through a person of trust, all but one of the delegates present subsequently agreed to be interviewed. After the interviews individuals also provided us with the contact details of some of their relatives, so enabling us to start snowballing. There was some reciprocity involved in our exchange with the president of the association, when he asked for a few words about the Congress to participants. Their organization had been asked by the Italian regional government to send a young delegate to the Congress, but they had failed to find anybody interested in going. Our Italian researcher thus became the delegate from the UK and so they felt some kind of responsibility towards her. The president of the regional organization also suggested that we use his wife's contacts since, because as he put it, 'women are more organized'. Whereas his main contacts were within the regional association, his wife was a member of a women's organization that included women from different regional and social backgrounds. She arranged for us to take part in a meeting of her organization. There, the women were somehow reluctant to take part in the study and none volunteered their contact details. Disappointed at how the evening was going, she and her sister started using their friendship with the other women to convince them to take part in the study. After that, we were able to interview several of them and also their husbands.

Two points can be drawn from this and other similar field experiences. First, it is of vital importance to establish personal connections, and this may involve spending time participating in meetings and events that are not always directly linked to the research being conducted. Members of regional and national associations and women's groups agreed to be interviewed after they had met us and talked in a setting that was familiar to them (albeit after a little mild 'arm twisting' in the case of Italian women's organizations). Second, there are benefits to be derived from using our informants' social capital. Although there are many advantages to this we soon became aware of, and uneasy about, using some of our informants' contacts and networks. Often we asked our informants, who operated in a 'gate-keeper' role, to provide us with further interviewees by drawing on their personal connections, and they sometimes put at our disposal the contacts derived from their central position within their communal or associational life to help us identify potential interviewees. They kindly used their position of trust and respectability to persuade others to take part in the study.

It is not, of course, possible or perhaps even desirable, to record and analyse all aspects of the research process, and much of this rich experience must remain with those who designed, organized and conducted the research. Experienced researchers, however, from any field in the humanities and social studies, will readily understand the silences or absences in any attempt to describe the research process. Nonetheless, we felt it useful to describe aspects of this experience in this chapter, partly because the research process in a work of this kind resonates with the very subject of analysis. And, as social researchers, we feel that we must be conscious of the debt we owe to individuals, families and communities; this carries a responsibility to adhere as closely as possible to the principles articulated by Weber and Myrdal as discussed earlier.

Conclusion

In this chapter we have set out some of the problems we had to face in constructing and conducting our empirical research on transnational families in a variety of local, national and transnational settings. The problems of interpreting the representations of transnational family lives will be seen as we approach particular issues in Part II of the book, and we will be referring back to the issues raised in these first chapters. However, before concluding this first part, it is necessary to give a general impression of the making of post-imperial British society as a result of immigration since the 1950s.

Note

1 Our third project concentrated on gaining an understanding of the utilization of social capital in households and family through the rituals of daily life as well as the specific stages of family and individual life cycles. This focus was encouraged by a suggestion from Gardner and Grillo (2002: 186) about Goulbourne's (1999) work on Caribbean transnational families: their suggestion was that attention to family ritual would strengthen his insistence that a key feature of Caribbean transnational families in Britain is their use of these links as part of their survival strategy in a hostile social environment. The attempt, however, was to test this with regard to other transnational families. We sought, therefore, in this project to focus on two communities with very different backgrounds in India – Punjabis and Goans. Our data consist mainly of observations of community

groups in London and participation-observations in Goa and the Punjab, and while we do not explicitly draw on these data in this book, the data have been useful to us in understanding the data from our Caribbean and Italian projects.

4   The politics of migration

Introduction

In the previous three chapters we focused on the background to the research on which this book is based and the theoretical and methodological issues that we faced in conducting our research on transnational families and communities. In particular, we located our core questions within the wider literature on migration and transnational families and outlined the key methodological issues we faced in developing our research and the conceptual debates about the social relations that shape the changing experiences of transnational families. Our main concern thus far has been on the wider conceptual and historical background to the research we carried out, with the aim of situating our work within the main bodies of research relevant to our own work. In this chapter we shift our focus to issues of migration that have helped to shape key aspects of British politics and society in the period since 1945, and which set the socio-political context for the analyses that follow in Part II of this book. This will clarify how migration conditions and influences families and communities, issues about diversity, and the mobilization of social capital, and will enable us to make important links with the range of issues and thematic concerns discussed in subsequent chapters.

Migration, politics and policy

The study of migration and the social and political issues that it gives rise to have expanded greatly since the 1990s. This has resulted in a noticeable growth of specialist courses, research centres and scholarly journals whose main focus is the interrelationship between migration and social and political change (Bauböck 2006; Guiraudon and Lahav 2007; Castles and Miller 2009). This growth has taken place, however, largely parallel to, rather than in a close dialogue with, the large body of work that developed from the 1960s onwards in Britain as well as other societies about the sociology of race and racism, migrant communities and forms of racial inequality and exclusion. There have been some attempts to link the various strands of analysis and to weave them together both conceptually as well as empirically (Castles 2000; Stasiulis and Ross 2006; Messina 2007). It remains by and large the case, however, that citizenship, migration and the inclusion and exclusion of minorities and migrants tend to be treated as largely discrete academic and political fields of interest. Although it is accepted that there are connections between these fields and links have been made, for example, between the study of migration and race relations, growing ethnic diversity and multiculturalism, and vice versa, the mechanisms through which these connections are actually worked through have only been partially the focus of substantive research (Aleinikoff 2002; Boswell 2007; Bloemraad *et al.* 2008). Rather, the tendency has been to analyse questions about migration separately from the study of race and ethnic relations.

Though there are good reasons for adopting such a focused approach a growing number of scholars have in recent years attempted to integrate studies of migration and racism with the analysis of the complexities of racial and ethnic diversity in contemporary societies. This is partly a result of the changing political and social climate, including evidence that questions about immigration, minority formation and citizenship are increasingly interrelated in terms of policy agendas and political mobilization. It is also to some extent the result of changing academic research agendas, as evidenced in the rapid growth of studies of multiculturalism, citizenship and religious as well as cultural diversity. The ongoing debates about the changing boundaries of national and transnational identities, the growth of what some authors have termed 'super diversity' and the assertion of cultural and religious identities are perhaps the most recent examples of this broader trend (Benhabib 2002; Bloemraad 2007; Vertovec 2007).

It is in this context that we embarked on the research that we cover in this book, and this is reflected in the ways that we framed the research around the interconnections between ethnicity, race and social capital in the everyday lives of transnational families. Rather than look at these processes in isolation our focus has been on the possible interconnections between them and their impact on contemporary British society. In particular we have sought to cover the changing forms of the experiences of minority communities and families during the current transformations which the wider British society has been going through. The core empirical focus of the case studies we conducted was precisely on the lived family experiences of migrant minority communities and their descendants.

Before moving on to discuss aspects of these contemporary trends in more substantive detail we discuss the historical context that helped to shape the present-day experiences of the minority communities that we cover in this study. In other words, we outline the historical background to the migration processes and patterns of settlement that has helped to condition minority formation in British society over the past 60 years.

Historical trends and processes

The history of migration to Britain and the creation of minority communities and institutions has been the subject of both historical and contemporary research. Much of this research has sought to provide an overview of both general patterns of migration and settlement as well as to situate the experiences of particular communities within this larger analytical frame that situates immigration in relation to popular ideas about race and minorities (Holmes 1988; Rich 1990).

This research has tended to see the history of immigration and minority formation as organized into three broad historical phases from the end of the nineteenth century to the present. In outline, the first phase lasted from the end of the nineteenth century to the beginning of the twentieth century and involved the arrival and settlement of Jewish migrants from Eastern Europe who had escaped the pogroms of the late nineteenth century. By 1914 the Jewish population in Britain had risen to around 300,000, which led to legislative measures, beginning in 1905 with the Aliens Act, that set limits on the numbers of immigrants who could enter Britain, and an increase in deportations (Solomos 2003; Kushner 2009). This was an important period in the formation of public policies about minorities and immigration within British society, and a period that saw the politicization of immigration and the articulation of anti-immigrant political ideologies, which were also often linked to ethno-racial ideologies.

At the same time Britain had small settlements of 'coloured people' and small numbers of 'coloured colonial citizens', including those who were resident over several generations and those arriving in the military or as seamen. These settlements were to be found in the older port cities, especially those associated with the Slave Trade – for example, Liverpool, Bristol and Cardiff – as well as London. These settlements numbered no more than perhaps 20,000, constituting a tiny percentage of the national population. There is clear evidence of racial discrimination in these towns and cities, but it was largely local and largely ignored at the national level (Harris 1988).

Perhaps the most important phase in the history of immigration can be found in the decades after 1945, which saw the arrival of migrants from the British colonies, particularly from the West Indies, India and Pakistan. This phase was to last until the late 1980s. It was in this period that a recognizable national politics around the question of immigration and race relation surfaced and in turn influenced the passage of legislation by successive governments from the 1960s to the 1970s. Public policies and debate about immigration during this period was focused specifically on the arrival of migrants from the Caribbean, India, Pakistan and other Commonwealth countries. Policies were developed in the period after 1962 to curtail migration from Commonwealth countries and brought to an end virtually all primary migration from the Caribbean and South Asia (Favell 2001; Goulbourne 1991; Bleich 2003).

The third phase, at the end of the twentieth century and the start of the twenty-first century, has focused on the question of new patterns of migration and particularly the arrival of asylum seekers and refugees. Legislation in the 1960s and 1970s had closed nearly all available routes for entering the country, with the exception of family reunions. By the 1990s and the early 2000s, however, the figure of the asylum seeker had gained prominence in public debates about migration to Britain. Conflict, political oppression, discrimination and abuses of human rights have all resulted in migration and increasing numbers of refugees and asylum seekers arriving in Britain and in the advanced economies of Europe and North America. Legislative responses to this have tried to control the numbers of asylum seekers entering Britain as well as to channel them into particular areas of British society through dispersal, exclusion from mainstream welfare provision and exclusion from the regular labour market (Bloch 2002; Schuster 2003).

For the communities that are the main focus of this study the period after 1945 was central to their experiences of migration and settlement. Immediately after the Second World War, faced with a serious labour shortage that could not be filled by Britain's traditional reserve army of labour, the Irish, the Labour Government decided to import some of the thousands of Europeans who had been displaced by war. They were given preference over Commonwealth citizens because, among other reasons, there was considerable prejudice against the recruitment of black colonial workers (Goulbourne 1998; Solomos 2003). Thus significant numbers of Europeans migrated and settled in Britain, particularly after the Second World War. This included 157,300 persons of Polish origin, around 75,000 persons who were displaced from their countries after the war and arrived on the European Volunteer Workers programme, around 8,300 Ukrainian prisoners of war, 5,000 Italians (who may have returned after their two-year contracts), and 85,000 refugees from Europe (Solomos 2003: 49–51). Between 1945 and 1951 approximately 70,000–100,000 people from the Republic of Ireland also settled in Britain.

Nonetheless, this limited supply was soon exhausted and from 1948 black Commonwealth citizens from the Caribbean and elsewhere arrived in Britain to meet the demand for labour. From this point on, the control of migration became a significant and continuing issue for Labour (and Conservative) Governments. It was an issue that became even more politicized and racialized after the riots in Nottingham and Notting Hill in 1958 (Pilkington 1988). Following the Notting Hill riots, concern focused on the problems caused by 'too many coloured immigrants in relation to housing, employment and crime', but also on the effect that black immigration would have on the 'racial character of the British people' (Solomos 2003: ch. 3). Although the 'race riots' in both Nottingham and Notting Hill were in essence attacks by local whites on black migrants, in both the media and public discourses they were explained through the lens of being an example of the racial tensions and conflicts that immigration was likely to lead to. The proposed solution for these problems was to restrict the migration of black Commonwealth citizens, though it was not until 1961 that legislation was presented to parliament restricting entry. The delay was due in part to legal and moral difficulties associated with restricting the entry of Commonwealth citizens to the 'Mother Country'. The 1962 Commonwealth Immigrants Act was introduced by the Conservatives, but shortly after taking office in 1964, the Labour Government under Harold Wilson issued a White Paper calling for stricter migration controls and signalled a growing convergence between Labour and the Conservatives on migration. The 1968 Commonwealth Immigrants Act introduced by Labour was explained in terms of either a response to public fears of black immigration or to economic interests that required a controlled and exploitable migrant labour force. However, Labour and Conservative Governments were not merely responsive, but had actively regulated and racialized immigration. In 1955–6, a policy of explicit control of black migration came close to being adopted by the Conservative Government, and the two Acts just referred to explicitly denied the automatic right to entry and abode to black and Asian British citizens (Carter *et al.* 1987; Rattansi 2005).

Migrant communities and racial discrimination

This linkage of immigration to the question of race has been a feature of political culture in Britain throughout the post-1945 period. From the early 1960s race relations policies in Britain have, in one way or another, been premised on the notion that the aims of public policy were: (i) to encourage the gradual integration of existing minorities by dealing with issues such as discrimination, education, social adjustment and welfare; (ii) to promote better community relations by stopping new immigration. This approach was based on the idea that the fewer immigrants, particularly ones that were visibly different in some manner, there were, the easier it would be to integrate them into the 'British way of life' and its social as well as cultural values. However, ongoing discrimination in education, employment and housing and troubled community relations has created a major dilemma for successive governments. Racist attacks on, and unrest within, migrant communities created an awareness that the question of racial discrimination had the potential to become a volatile political issue.

This potential existed in both majority and minority communities. There was the negative response of some of the majority white population to the arrival of migrants in what were perceived to be sizeable numbers, although Britain at that stage was still a country of net emigration. At the same time there was the frustration of ethnic minority communities who were excluded from equal participation in British society by discrimination in the labour and housing markets, along with related processes of social and political exclusion. Both these issues were perceived as potential sources of conflict that the government had to manage and control.

While there had been a great deal of discussion and debate around these issues during the previous two decades, the first attempts to deal with the potential for racial conflict and to tackle racial discrimination can be traced back to the 1960s and continued into the 1970s. They took two basic forms. The first involved the setting up of agencies to deal with the problems faced by black migrants and to help the white communities understand the migrants. The setting up of the National Committee for Commonwealth Immigrants in the early 1960s was symptomatic of this integrationist policy agenda. It led later in the 1960s to the setting up of the Community Relations Commission and local Community Relations Councils, whose main objective was to improve relations between majority and minority communities.

The second stage of the policy response, signalled by the passage of the 1965, 1968 and 1976 Race Relations Acts, was premised on the notion that the state should attempt to ban discrimination on the basis of race, colour or ethnic origin through legal sanctions. The latter Act also created public regulatory agencies charged with the task of promoting greater equality of opportunity, particularly the Commission for Racial Equality, which oversaw the implementation of race relations policies from 1977 to 2006 (Commission for Racial Equality 2006). These measures were supposed to provide equal access to employment, education, housing and public facilities generally. Successive governments stated their commitment to this broad objective, and developed policies that promised to tackle various aspects of direct and indirect racial discrimination, to promote greater equality of opportunity and to remedy other social disadvantages suffered by black minority communities in British society. According to a number of studies carried out during both the 1980s and 1990s these promises remain unfulfilled (Modood *et al.* 1997).

For successive governments, both Conservative and Labour, the need for tight controls on immigration was taken as given. During the 1960s and 1970s the legislative framework for controlling immigration, particularly from the New Commonwealth, became a key component of policy in this field. From a broader historical vantage point therefore it is important to remember that since the 1960s the Labour Party has endorsed the need for immigration controls, and the 1968 Act, driven through parliament at speed in the face of further migration from East Africa, was in line with Conservative migration policy. Although at key points the two parties diverged somewhat as to the specific nature of immigration policy and in the manner in which legislation was to be implemented, the Labour Party differed only to a limited extent from the mainstream of the Conservative Party. This relative consensus in policy agendas between the two main political parties was a feature of the whole period from the mid-1970s to the late 1980s (Solomos 2003).

During the long period of Conservative domination from 1979 to 1997, however, there was some divergence in orientation between Labour and the Conservatives. Part of the reason for this divergence can be seen in terms of the shifts within the Conservative Party on questions about race and immigration that became evident under the Thatcher Governments from 1979 onwards. The hardening of Conservative rhetoric on race as exemplified by Margaret Thatcher's 'swamping speech' and Norman Tebbit's 'cricket test' was an important element of the neo-Conservative ideology of the right wing of the party (Ansell 1997; Smith 1994). Throughout the Conservatives' 18 years in office there had been numerous calls for the strengthening of the 1976 Race Relations Act. The Commission for Racial Equality made detailed submissions supporting these calls, and research highlighted the limits of the 1976 Act, limits that had become pronounced as early as the 1980s. However, the Conservatives preferred to concentrate on migration controls, arguing that if migration – and hence the size of minority populations – were controlled, there would be no major 'race problem'. The Conservatives introduced a series of Acts designed to exclude migrants originating from some countries, but not others (those granted work permits, admitted to seek work or a variation to their visas to enable them to seek work have largely come from the white Commonwealth and the USA). The first of these was the 1981 British Nationality Act, which created further categories of citizen with different rights of abode and effectively deprived British citizens of (mostly) Asian origin of the right to live in Britain (Goulbourne 1991; Cohen 1994).

The divergence between the two parties seemed to become more pronounced during the early 1990s as the issue of refugees and asylum seekers moved higher onto the Conservatives political agenda. Following the fall of the Berlin Wall, the old Cold War certainties and stability disappeared. As a result of the war in Yugoslavia, the number of asylum seekers increased significantly, and though they were not of the same magnitude as those seeking asylum in Germany, the Conservative Government responded with very restrictive legislation and very hostile language. In 1993, the Conservative Government brought in the Asylum and Immigration Appeal Act, which was the first piece of primary legislation to deal with asylum, and in 1996 the Asylum and Immigration Act, which removed asylum seekers from the benefit system and shifted financial responsibility to local authorities (Hussain 2001).

By the early 2000s, however, this divergence was to some extent replaced by a convergence on the part of both the main political parties on a policy agenda about race and immigration that focused on the possible dangers of immigration and increasing ethnic, religious and cultural diversity to the fabric of social cohesion. This is a point we return to at the end of this chapter.

Migrant communities, radicalization and politics

The 1950s to the 2000s saw an increasingly explicit racialization of immigration in which issues of race came to dominate the political agenda, and the popular perception of what immigration was all about in this period. There was a shift in official policy from decrying an open and explicit discussion of race in the debate on immigration, and allowing it to be shaped by the economic needs of the country, to the view that there should be explicit consideration of the race of immigrants, especially those of African-Caribbean, and Indian or Pakistani background, in framing national policy. There was also more of an acceptance of the argument that the 'genuine fears' (often a proxy for racial prejudice) of the indigenous white population should be taken into account in deciding how many such immigrants to allow into the country. Once a strict limit on such immigration has been achieved, attention turned towards the residents as a source of concern.

The racialization of immigration can be traced back to the 1950s and 1960s. This point is highlighted in much of the literature on the politics of immigration in this period. There is disagreement, however, over how it came about, and the consequences of state policies (Goulbourne 1998; Miles and Phizacklea 1984; Pilkington 1988). Robert Miles and Annie Phizacklea, for example, see it as the result of the pressure group activities of a small group of racist politicians, and members of the white public, especially in the Midlands, who fomented fear over competition for limited resources such as jobs, education, housing and health, in the context of British capitalism's inability to meet the needs of the vast majority of workers (Miles and Phizacklea 1984). In this interpretation these racist groups were able to influence the attitudes of the white population generally, and the actions of significantly placed politicians and government, by forcing the issue of race to the front of the immigration debate, out of all proportion to its relevance, and maintaining it there. Once there, it has not been dislodged. Miles and Phizacklea oscillate on the role of the white British population. On the one hand they see them as the victims of the activities of a small number of white racists, inside and outside British Government. But later on in their book *White Man's Country* they represent a majority of whites in the nation as being a major part of the 'anti-coloured movement' that forced the issue of immigration controls on the basis of race onto the political agenda.

Authors such as Sivanandan, on the other hand, see the racialization of British immigration policies as the result of the activities of the state, in the context of its functions as the manager of the needs of British capital (Sivanandan 1982, 1990). In describing the 1950s and 1960s, Sivanandan argues that the state sought first to entice labour from the colonies to meet the labour needs of capital, and then to restrict coloured immigrants when British capitalism was unable to provide enough jobs for all the workers in the nation. Sivanandan sees successive types of immigration control as a means of subordinating such 'coloured immigrants' and, more generally, non-British immigrants and asylum seekers, into the lowest subservient roles of labour, particularly those kinds no longer desired by indigenous white workers.

The 1948 British Nationality Act gave the right to enter, work and settle in Britain to all colonial and Commonwealth citizens. This is what was already happening in practice but the Act sought to formalize these practices. Immigration policies during this period were framed by, and dominated by, 'open door' policies, that is, the idea that all subjects of the United Kingdom and colonies should have the right of entry to work and settle in the UK. The evidence for this period indicates that actual immigration flows tended to follow the economic demands of employers.

The 1949 Royal Commission on Population identified a significant shortage of labour in Britain and said the country might need to encourage 140,000 young immigrants each year, and that it would also require considerable expenditure on housing and social services (Miles and Phizacklea 1984: 24). In June 1948, the ship *Empire Windrush* arrived in Tilbury docks (see, Phillips and Phillips 1998) with over 400 British West Indian subjects and over 50 Polish women. This is usually heralded as the start of so-called 'large-scale' West Indian immigration, and arguably signalled the beginning of the multicultural society in Britain (see, Goulbourne 1998).

The 'open door' policy prevailed and immigration flows continued to closely correspond with the needs of employers. Select employers – British Rail, the National Health Service, London Transport – made deliberate, targeted efforts to recruit labour from the Commonwealth. These employers were responsible for the direct recruitment of thousands of 'coloured colonial subjects'. Domestic policies included limited initiatives to aid immigrants to find housing and jobs, and it was more likely to be voluntary associations who provided such services and advice. There were also very limited language provisions, and most immigrants had to find their own way, accommodation, and so forth.

There was evidence of some hostility towards such immigrants – colour bars in pubs and night clubs, fights in pubs, including, especially, the 1958 riots in Notting Hill, London and Nottingham, which largely consisted of young white men attacking West Indian men, though, as noted, the riots were portrayed in the media as 'race riots' (Pilkington 1988). The increasing numbers of West Indians arriving in the nation, as compared with the tiny settlements of such people previously, along with the sparse but highly publicized incidents of conflict, put the issue of 'coloured immigration' constantly in the front pages of the media. And in the debates in the House of Commons over the nature and form of immigration, and the provisions being made to accommodate it, there was intensity and volatility. By 1961 a Gallup National Poll indicated that 73 per cent of the British population wanted immigration control, and that they were thinking primarily of control against 'coloured colonial immigrants'. Many politicians publicly voiced alarm about this immigration and several voiced support for immigration controls. The result was the 1962 Commonwealth Immigration Act introduced by the Conservative Government which introduced work vouchers for immigrants from the Commonwealth as the main method of restricting immigration.

Alongside the pressure to control and regulate immigration there was a shift of attention to the 'second generation', children of migrants who were seen as a potential source of concern. By the 1970s, there was a large and growing population of indigenous youth of West Indian and Indian or Pakistani origins who were having relatively tough times in the labour market. Youth of West Indian origin were seen as faring the worse, and there was concern about the social and political consequences of allowing young people from minority backgrounds to become ever more marginalized from the mainstream of society (Solomos 1991). These popular fears merged in the 1970s with wider concerns about street crime and urban dislocation. In particular, in cities such as Birmingham and London there was a concern that the 'second generation' of young West Indians were drifting into a marginal role in society, often typified by concerns about their involvement in street crimes such as 'mugging' and increasing contact with the police and the criminal justice system (Hall *et al.* 1978).

It should also be noted that in the 1970s and 1980s anti-racism grew as an important political ideology, linked to popular campaigns with an emphasis on confronting racism, and of highlighting the relationship between racism and other social inequalities. Such initiatives were premised on the need to tackle both the root cause of racism and exclusion and to develop policies for the inclusion of minority communities within society on an equal basis. Such initiatives received support from local authorities that were often at the forefront of developing policies dealing with such issues as housing and education in relation to minority communities.

In 1979 Margaret Thatcher became prime minister in Britain; before the general election she made the famous 'swamping statement' about the impact of immigration on British culture. Thatcher made it clear that her government was going to take a hard line on any stridency by immigrants to demand their rights, and when there were widespread riots across the nation in 1981 and later on in 1985 her first response was to condemn the riots as an outcome of criminal activity and lawlessness. Despite her reaction, the Scarman Report on the 1981 riots found evidence of racial disadvantage everywhere in England but said the police were not institutionally racist. Scarman called for more efforts to tackle racial discrimination – but few were forthcoming (Scarman 1981, 1985; Benyon and Solomos 1987, 1988).

Current agendas and debates

Policy agendas about immigration and race had by the late 1990s become focused on the twin objectives of using governmental interventions to promote both community cohesion and recognition of the cultural and ethnic diversity of British society. This was particularly the focus of the first New Labour administration under Tony Blair from 1997 to 2001, a period that saw renewed commitment to addressing racial injustice and constructing a multi-ethnic society. Such commitment was evidenced both by the publication of the Macpherson Report in 1999 and other initiatives that helped to shape public discourses in this field (Macpherson 1999; McGhee 2008).

Significant discussions and many policy initiatives continued in the 1990s, as the populations from the Commonwealth became more and more indigenous. With the break-up of the Soviet Union, and with problems of poverty and political terror in many nations, Britain saw its immigrant population becoming more and more white and European, with those who were not white more likely to arrive in the form of asylum seekers. In the immediate aftermath of the 1997 General Election the most noticeable initiatives were connected to questions about race relations. New Labour attempted to put 'clear blue water' between itself and the Conservative Party by emphasizing its commitment to social justice for racial minorities (Schuster and Solomos 2004). It introduced some important initiatives, including the Stephen Lawrence Inquiry and the subsequent Macpherson Report in 1999, the 1998 Crime and Disorder Act, the 2000 Race Relations (Amendment) Act, and it also seemed to take on board some of the arguments of the independent Parekh report, *The Future of Multi-Ethnic Britain*. These were only the most high-profile initiatives, but they signalled what seemed to be a 'radical turn' in government policy on race relations.

The publication in February 1999 of the Macpherson Report into the murder of Stephen Lawrence gave the Home Office the necessary impetus to revisit the 1976 Race Relations Act and seemed to herald a new commitment to racial equality and justice. In many ways the report can be said to contain little that is new, either in conceptual analysis or in policy agenda setting. It is a rather mixed bag of recommendations based on scholarly research over the previous two decades and policy recommendations across a whole range of issues. However, the report gave rise to a high level of public attention on publication and in the period that followed. An important element of its influence can be seen in terms of the fact that it covers a much broader canvas in its recommendations than the actual events surrounding the murder of Stephen Lawrence and the police response to the murder. It includes recommendations, for example, about general policies on race relations, racism, education and social policy. This is in some ways part of its strength, but it also means that in judging its political effectiveness we have to be aware of the range of policy arenas that are discussed in the report and the likely political outcomes.

There seems little doubt that the Macpherson Report has had an important symbolic impact in shaping New Labour's thinking about the question of institutionalized racism, but its impact in terms of practical policy change in the medium term remains to be assessed. The preliminary evidence since 1999 indicates that at least some key elements of the report are being implemented, particularly as the government seeks to show that it is taking the question of 'institutional racism' seriously within its own institutions, such as the police and the civil service. Recent research by the then Commission for Racial Equality has indicated that there has been some progress within central government departments, such as the Home Office, in developing programmes to further the recruitment, retention and promotion of minority staff. In particular, the 2000 Race Relations (Amendment) Act may prove to be an important tool in ensuring that public bodies take on board the 'duty to promote' racial equality.

The 2000 Act, which came into force on 1 December 2001, enforces on public authorities a new general statutory duty to promote racial equality. The expectation embodied in the Act is that public authorities will take action to:

- prevent acts of race discrimination before they occur
- ensure that in performing their public functions they should 'have due regard to the need to eliminate unlawful racial discrimination, and to promote equality of opportunity and good relations between persons of different racial groups'.

While the 2000 Act was generally welcomed as a positive step by many of those concerned with how best to tackle racial discrimination and exclusion, there was, nonetheless, some disappointment that the Act did not take up all the recommendations made by the Commission for Racial Equality for strengthening the 1976 Race Relations Act. Perhaps the most telling section of the Act was Section 19, which excluded immigration and asylum and refuge from the remit of the Act.

In the period since 2001 there has been a recognizable shift to a much harder position in public policy discourses about ethnic minorities and the wider politics of race. In the context of more popular media coverage this is signalled by recurring stories and concerns about a 'crisis of multiculturalism' and fears about a drift towards segregation and a lack of social cohesion in urban communities as well as in the wider society. This transformation in discourses about race and multiculturalism can be traced to a number of interrelated processes.

The first of these processes took place between May and July 2001 and involved clashes between gangs of white and British Asian youths in a number of northern British towns, notably Oldham, Burnley, Blackburn and Bradford. These clashes had a number of both local and national causes and resulted in scores of arrests, hundreds of injuries and considerable damage to property. A number of inquiries into the events highlighted the role of social and economic dislocation in the various towns as well as trends towards separation between majority white communities and the largely British Asian communities in these towns (Cantle 2001; Denham 2001; Ouseley 2001).

The second process was set in motion by the terrorist attacks on the World Trade Center in New York on 9/11. The attacks on New York were carried out by a Muslim terrorist group based on a transnational network of activists, but it is also clear that indirectly they have had a major impact on debates about immigration and race relations (Calhoun *et al.* 2002; Foner 2005; Rodriguez 2008). The terrorist attacks on the London transport system in July 2005, which were carried out by young British Muslims, gave added weight to the fears and concerns generated by 9/11 and played an important role in changing the terms of public discourse about race and the position of minorities in British society. In the wake of the 9/11 and 7/7 terrorist attacks and international concerns over national security, migration is increasingly framed in relation to terrorism, crime, unemployment and religious fundamentalism rather than offering new opportunities for European societies in relation to cosmopolitanism and national economic development

The third process that has shaped the current social and political agenda has been the renewed focus on questions about migration, whether in the form of new patterns of migration or in the form of forced migrants and asylum seekers and refugees. In Britain this focus was symbolized throughout the late 1990s and early 2000s by continual media coverage and policy interventions about asylum seekers and refugees and concerns that growing numbers of economic migrants were likely to seek to move to Britain. This renewal of interest in questions about immigration has done much to influence both public policies and also the wider societal debate about the impact of migrants on the wider society.

Migration impacts on a range of processes, including economies, development, politics, culture, community, family and household relations. Globalization, global inequality, conflicts, oppression, and technological advances in transportation, media and communications will ensure that global migration will continue and that migrants will hold multiple identities as well as obligations to kinship groups in their country of origin and elsewhere. Migration has resulted in the formation of new communities that are developing a strong tradition of migration. In the case of the UK, numbers within established migrant groups from the Caribbean, India, Pakistan and Bangladesh have increased, mainly due to internal natural growth rather than new migration. At the time of the 1991 census, 5.5 per cent of the population described themselves as coming from an ethnic group other than white, increasing to 7.9 per cent of the population by the 2001 census. Britain has also seen an increase in new migrants and the formation of new migrant groups from countries without prior links to the UK. This has included refugees and asylum seekers from all over the world as well as migrant workers with both regular and irregular immigration statuses.

This renewal of public debate about immigration is not purely a British phenomenon. Migration is high on the international policy agenda due to the increasing scales of international migration as well as the challenges and opportunities that this can present. The precise numbers of international migrants is unknown, but in 1990 there were 80 million migrants and this had increased to 175 million, or 2.9 per cent of the global population, by 2000. Of these global migrants, just under 10 per cent are refugees (Castles 2004, 2007). Within this evolving international environment the experience of Britain highlights both the relevance of migration as an important social and political issue and the likelihood that it will remain on the agenda as a key phenomenon for the coming decades.

Conclusion

The interrelationship between policies on immigration, integration and community relations has been a recurring theme in research and scholarship for some time. In this chapter we have focused on situating the processes of migration and settlement that have shaped the experiences of British society of the communities that we are looking at in the context of our substantive analysis in the rest of the volume. A core issue we have been concerned with in this context has been the process that has shaped the changing experiences of ethnic minority communities over the past half century and more. In focusing on this issue we have touched on questions about the changes that we have seen in policies and agendas about immigration and minority communities over the past few decades. We have emphasized the often contradictory nature of policies and agendas in the post-1945 period, although there is by now clear recognition that Britain is an increasingly multicultural society that needs to develop forms of identity and belonging that respect both individual rights and the identities of particular groups and communities, while a new or transformed British identity or identities emerge. We now move on to some substantive chapters that cover key facets of the studies of transnational families that framed the empirical components of our research. Our main concern in these chapters is the analysis of the intersections between ethnicity, families and social capital in the formation of lived experiences within transnational families.

Part II

Living and coping across boundaries

Part II

Living and coping across boundaries

5 Migrants, offspring and settlement

Introduction

In this and the following chapters, we draw on the data we collected in Britain, the Caribbean and Italy to analyse specific aspects of the transnational lives of families in Britain. We outline how Caribbean immigrants and their offspring described the patterns of their settlement and integration into British society, and how they explained continuing kinship ties 'back home' that facilitated these processes. With respect to Italians, the chapter draws on the existing literature to give a skeletal account of their settlement patterns, particularly in the post-Second World War years. The chapter therefore also addresses whether and how subsequent generations followed the patterns established by their parents and in some cases grandparents. We take into account the wider social networks that members of these new communities forged in the process of establishing new homes in Britain, as well as friendships within same-ethnic and cross-ethnic boundaries.

Community settlement and formation

Following the politics that accompanied the process of immigration described in the last chapter, it was not surprising that migrants in the post-Second World War period settled in particular parts of the country. In the main, these were where employment and residential opportunities existed, and from where many members of the indigenous population were moving, to relocate in the more pleasant environments created as a result of the rebuilding of war-torn inner-cities. There is little to be gained by repeating here the statistical evidence of the demographic distribution of Caribbean migrants and their offspring in Britain since the Second World War (see, for example, Patterson 1965; Owen 1994, 2006). Rather, what is necessary is to highlight the subjective perceptions of our interviewees about questions of where to settle. For example, migrant mothers were nearly all working and needed to establish networks to assist with childcare. They therefore found it providential to live in neighbourhoods where there were already a number of Caribbeans living and where affordable childcare services could be accessed. In reflecting on the early days of entry and settlement, many mothers pointed out that living in such neighbourhoods enabled their children to maintain a degree of contact with their cultural roots and identity. Later generations also believed that what had developed to become neighbourhoods with a degree of ethnic specificity provided transmission of cultural values across generations.

Our interviews with Caribbean offspring also suggested that these young adults were influenced by their parents' settlement patterns. Their parents' initial patterns of settlement determined children's choice of neighbourhoods in their adulthood, and the majority of young people grew up in inner-city neighbourhoods and within working-class households. Consequently, many of these offspring have experienced limited geographical and social mobility. Many of our respondents, for example, had never lived outside the area where they were born and as young adults they either continued to live at home with their parents or within adjacent neighbourhoods and less than 30 minutes' travelling time to their parents' homes. This is particularly interesting when we compare them with their parents, who migrated thousands of miles away from their family and friends in search of better social and economic opportunities and among whom there were also migrants who had experienced serial migration before settling in the UK. These young people had therefore strongly invested in regional ties or identities, such as proclaiming themselves to be a Londoner, a Mancunian or a Brummie, and many of them expressed a general reluctance to live beyond their own specific communities in Britain. They celebrated these specific regional identities, whilst also sometimes disclaiming allegiance or loyalty to national British or English identities. Adrian, a Londoner powerfully expressed this view in reply to a question about his identity in Britain; he told us that he was

> not English, no way would I call myself that, but I would say London, I'm definitely a Londoner. That's what I would call 'home'. That's where I want to come home to. I really love London and the way it's made up of different people. I couldn't imagine living anywhere else
>
> (Adrian, interview location: London, November 2003)

Many respondents perceived black neighbourhoods as a basis for political activities, collective mobilization, and an affirmation of their ethnic identities. In these communities there were areas of social life that reflected specific ethnic and racial characteristics, such as black night clubs and pubs; black hairdressers and barbers; restaurants and shops selling Caribbean food; theatres and exhibitions focusing on black cultural events; licensed and unlicensed radio stations; and of course, parlours with hair products, music, and so forth. For young people these neighbourhoods represented identifiable items that they could consume and physical spaces where they could engage in activities that demonstrated their racial and ethnic identities. In many cases, these young people used these neighbourhoods to draw ethnic and racial boundaries characterized by 'us' (black/Caribbean) and 'them' (white/English) as well as to build bonds and trust in what they saw as Caribbean communities. They tended to hold strong views about their communities and often pointed to the advantages as well as disadvantages of where they lived in terms of resources, perceptions of crime, safety and so forth. For Denise it was the convenience of her location that pleased her most:

I like Seven Sisters. Mostly it's quite central, it's not too far from the station, so I can do a quick run, in five minutes, to the station, if I'm really running late. The shops are just round the corner so I can run out and buy things at the last minute. This morning I felt like doing fried plantain for breakfast and I pulled my tracksuit to go out and I was there and back in 5 minutes. What I don't like is sometimes you get loud people, like noise on the road, like neighbours, and people just disturbing your kind of privacy, you know, they'd be nosey. And coming home late at night, sometimes, and you get people bothering you, you know, but you get that anywhere, and if you know, well I know how to handle yourself so I don't let it bother me, I don't feel unsafe in this area.

(Denise, interview location: London, April 2004)

An understanding of Caribbean communities must be situated within the wider context of social exclusion or racial discrimination. Emerging out of, and in response to, these experiences, black communities have developed strong bonds and activities to combat racism and exclusion. The idea that 'you have to get out to get on' and achieve upward social mobility (Holland *et al.* 2007) did not appear to reflect the views and experiences of some Caribbean respondents. Rather, they viewed their neighbourhoods as a 'safe haven' against the harsh daily realities of racial discrimination. They considered that the sense of security and cultural belongingness provided by their neighbourhoods acted as a platform from which social progress and social mobility could be built. In other words, they appeared to agree with Halpern's (2005: 262) suggestion that 'bonds between different ethnic groups may grow more strongly when those groups also maintain a strong internal sense of identity and bonding social capital'. In this respect, it would appear that these young people's strong bonding social capital acted as a precursor to bridging social capital across ethnic groups, as Carleen's forthright statement suggests:

I have no time for black people who don't want to know about their history or try to cut themselves off from the black community because they think they're somehow better. As far as I'm concerned they're lost and don't know who they are. How can you move forward if you don't know where you're coming from and you don't know your culture? I'm determined to have a successful career but it doesn't mean I'll cut myself off [from the black community] like some people do. I need to stay and help and bring others up behind me so they can see it's possible to be black and successful in life. My mentor is a top black barrister. Why I really admire her is [because] she went to a local comprehensive school like me. My close friends are black but I also have very good friends who are Malaysian, white, English and Suisse-German. And when they tell me about their cultures, I tell them about my Jamaican culture and history. It always surprises them because they assume we have no culture.

(Carleen, interview location: London, December 2003)

Sam in Birmingham echoed these sentiments when he said that

my parents always showed me my culture and we live in an area where there are lots of black people that have lived here for over 50 years. So, I have a strong sense of who I am as a black woman .... I live in a black neighbour-hood. People who don't come from here think it's an area with crime, drugs and poverty but living here I see lots of good things that go on. I make a point to share that with people who don't know any better.

(Sam, interview location: Birmingham, December 2003)

The bonding ties that contribute to the young people's emotional and psychological well-being were facilitated by their involvement and participation in ethnic-specific community associations, such as black-led church groups, youth groups and supplementary schools. They tended to have a strong sense of obligation and responsibility to be role models for Caribbean children in their communities; there was also a keenness to 'give back' to their communities that they felt had supported them to achieve what they had in the world.

The sense of safety and well-being experienced from being embedded in ethnic-specific communities or neighbourhoods does not, however, entirely enable people to overcome all obstacles placed in their way. Too strong a bonding to specific neighbourhoods and ethnic ties may indeed hinder individuals and groups in other areas of social life. A bonding that is too strong has the potential to restrict them from accessing resources outside their specific communities. Marion Orr's (1999) study of black communities in the USA examined this issue in relation to educational progression and achievement of black children living in working-class communities. Orr argued that whilst black community organizations had been suc-cessful in collectivizing and campaigning against racism and racial inequalities in schools, these organizations were largely ineffective in enlisting the cooperation of mainstream institutions which had greater resources that could benefit the black community. A similar situation exists in some British-Caribbean communities (see, for example, Gann 1998; also, Goring 2004).

A second argument posed by Orr (1999) was that inter-generation poverty was reproduced in working-class black neighbourhoods by young people them-selves because of their willingness to remain in their poorly resourced physical neighbourhoods and communities. These young people thereby chose not to go to well-resourced schools in white geographical areas, where they would have a greater chance of educational success and upward social mobility. In speaking to young people in British cities about factors that influenced their choice of higher education institutions many stated that this was determined by their desire to stay close to home. They generally chose local universities in black and urban areas where there was a sizeable body of black students and shied away from universities that may be better resourced (and may provide them with better opportunities) but would take them out of their 'comfort zones'. David made it clear to us that

[I] was offered two university places at East London University and Lancaster to study mechanical engineering. At first I was wanted to go to Lancaster, it has one of the best reputations for the course. What put me off was the place itself. I didn't see a black face. At the Open Day I'm the only black person. I kept thinking 'where are all the black people'. I saw a few Chinese students but they were overseas students. They didn't mix and they kept to themselves. It was a really white place and I didn't feel I belonged. The lecturers I met in the department were all white. I think the tutors were a bit intimidated by this 6ft 3ins black guy. I thought to myself 'I can't live here for 4 years. It's too white'. I wouldn't be able to settle down and that would affect my work. I'd always be running back to London or Leeds, just to see some black faces and feel comfortable. So I decided London was the place for me.

Q: Do you have any regrets about your choice?

A: No, not at all. No regrets. I'm happy and comfortable at college. We have all races and nationality on my course, lots of Blacks and Asians, lots of students from all over the world and we all get along. I don't stand out.

(David, interview location: London, January 2004)

David graduated from university with First Class Honours, and he attributed his success to the feeling that he was able to study in a comfortable and supportive environment, and where being a black student was not an issue. He was able to develop a strong peer and friendship network of black and minority ethnic students that supported him in his learning, which he felt would not have been available to him if he had accepted the other university place offered to him in a predominately white area with few black and minority ethnic students. The sense of belonging-ness he felt helped him to focus his energies on his studies. David's case was not exceptional, and the desire of some Caribbean young people to be embedded within their communities (even if this may be detrimental to their own personal success) must be understood within the wider context of social exclusion, which in turn encourages a desire for cultural belongingness.

The attachment to place, whether in England or in the Caribbean, was a painful aspect of the lives of the migrant generation themselves, particularly as they came to their twilight years. The question of return will be the subject of a later chapter, but it is worth noting at this point how worrying this can be for families. For example, Delia, a wife and grandmother, told us that she and her husband

had it all planned out, we've picked out our plot [of land] and its just waiting for us to starting building on it …. Lloyd [husband] is impatient to get out there and start building but I'm dragging my heels because what am I going out there for? My family is here. I don't want to be so far away from my children and grandchildren, they're my life now. I would be bored and lost without them. Its alright for Lloyd because men they're different, they don't have the same bond with the children like us women. … Whilst the dream is nice, the reality would be different and I'd feel so terrible being so far away

Q: Have you considered spending part of the year out there?

A: I don't think our pensions would stretch to allow us to come home regularly, and our savings we need to live on and emergencies, I'm not sure if the kids could afford to keep coming to see us … I think I'll stay here and I'm more needed here. Lloyd can go if he wants ... maybe when the grandchildren are older then I'll think about going if God spares life and my health is good

(Delia, interview location: London, January 2005)

Some migrants at this late stage of their lives decided to separate, with the men returning and the women staying on in England to be close to their children and grandchildren. Couples who could afford it travelled frequently between the two points, but it was noticeable that there were several men who had returned without their wives, and this appeared to reflect levels of commitments to children, grandchildren, as well as respective places of birth and settlement across the Atlantic world.

Italians have been in Britain as long as or longer than most minority ethnic communities, but perhaps because of their relative invisibility as indigenous Europeans and their numbers, their settlement patterns are less commented upon than those of visible communities, such as Caribbeans. While, therefore, we have drawn on the views of our Caribbean interviewees to describe aspects of settlement, we want here to give a more objective account of where Italians settled in Britain. As we draw upon the accounts of Italian migrants and their offspring in this and subsequent chapters, their own views of commitment to place and the formation of communities and neighbourhoods in Britain will become clearer.

In the years before the Second World War, impoverished northern Italian peasants migrated to London as itinerant workers engaged in a variety of activities ranging from street music to semi-skilled and skilled craft work (Colpi 1991: 40). The most notable craftsmen of this period were the *figurinai* (makers and sellers of small statuettes), the *terrazzo* (mosaic) workers and the *arrotini* (knife-grinders). The fathers of the northern Italians whom we interviewed were *arrotini*. Some of the migrants moved into the catering sector, first as itinerant workers selling chestnuts in winter and ice cream in summer, then as owners of small family businesses where they gained some success. They also started to move from London, seizing opportunities to open businesses elsewhere in the country. This phase came to a traumatic end at the beginning of the Second World War, with the closure of several Italian businesses and the internment of hundreds of Italians as suspected enemies (Palmer 1977; Colpi 1991).

A new type of Italian migration resumed after the war. These new migrants no longer originated from the mountainous regions of the north but rather from some of the most deprived areas of the south. Unlike the earlier wave these newcomers did not come through chain migration but arrived through labour-recruiting schemes set up by British firms in collaboration with the Italian Government in order to cover areas of labour shortage (King 1977; Tubito and King 1996; Colucci 2002). Rather than joining their predecessors in London and in the other areas of old 'little Italys' such as Manchester or Edinburgh, these new migrants settled near their new workplaces, in medium-sized industrial towns such as Bedford, Peterborough, Loughborough, Bletchley, Nottingham, Coventry, Sheffield and in the South Wales steel towns (Tubito and King 1996).

The largest concentration of Italians in Britain occurred in Bedford. The first cohort arrived in 1951, recruited from a centre near Naples by the London Brick Company (King 1977; King and King 1977; Colucci 2002), and by the late 1970s they were estimated at 8,000, representing the largest immigrant group in the city and 10 per cent of the Bedford population. The men started on four-year contracts in the brick industry and initially lived in hostels set up by their employers. Gradually they moved to rented properties near the town centre and were joined by their families. Men often continued to work in the brick industry but some moved to less strenuous blue-collar jobs or opened small shops. Like Caribbeans, the women had a high level of labour market participation. They worked in hospitals, domestic service and the food and electronic industries. In the 1970s, the confectionery company Meltis alone employed 600 Italian women in Bedford (King 1977; King and King 1977). Through hard work and frugal lives, many Italians managed to accumulate some savings and were able to buy their own homes in Bedford and in the other towns where they had settled. After the closure of the Naples recruitment centre in 1957, the London Brick Company continued to recruit Italians through their workers' personal networks, thereby favouring chain migration (King 1977).

Some researchers have noted the differences between these pre-war and post-war Italian communities (see, Cavallaro 1981; Colpi 1991; Fortier 2000). The former have been seen as well integrated into British society, whereas the latter are usually depicted as particularly attached to their own traditions, living confined lives with their families, their village groups and the Catholic church, and with social interactions rarely extending beyond kin members and co-villagers.

Our respondents belonged to both these groups. The southern Italians we interviewed and who had migrated in the 1950s and 1960s formed close-knit communities where rigid norms and values were maintained and where there were strong internal social control. Economically, this group was relatively successful, managing to buy small terraced houses and helping financially to set up their children by paying for their expensive weddings and with buying their first homes. At the time of our interviews, their children worked mainly in clerical, hairdressing and mechanical jobs, but few joined the professions. The migrant generation tended not to wish their children to pursue further education since the family's plan was to save enough money as quickly as possible and return to Italy. University in the UK was seen as a waste of time and money, and parents preferred their children to start working soon after leaving compulsory education and contribute to the family budget; most resources were invested in Italy (in areas such as Ribera), especially in houses.

Migrants' offspring from this group were expected to live close to their parents, but some moved away to new suburban neighbourhoods and travelled to their families. Some young people also moved away from home to study or work but, especially in the case of women, this was generally seen in very negative terms, as we will see in a later chapter. It is important to note that rather than being seen as a sign of upward social mobility these moves were seen as deserting family and community responsibilities.

The second group of Italian settlement patterns in the UK is characterized by the Trentini in London. Those migrating from the Trentino region after the war were continuing a tradition that had started at the beginning of the century. By the 1950s and 1960s, the Italian 'community' in London had dispersed from their original centre in the Clerkenwell area, and entered the knife-grinding occupation. By the 1950s and 1960s there were small workshops where the knives were brought to be sharpened for butchers, restaurateurs and hoteliers. This occupation has survived and Trentini came to own modern workshops, some employing several workers. Those migrating in the 1950s and 1960s were housed and employed by the previous migrants. Women of the older group set up informal bed and breakfast accommodation in their homes, where they cooked and washed for the new wave of village men. These men stayed in these houses until they were married, some with village girls and some with English girls. These living arrangements were also common with Caribbean migrants during this period.

Whereas the early migrants had settled close to the Italian church in Clerkenwell, the post-war migrant group settled predominantly in south London and had as their reference point the Italian church on Brixton Road. For example, at one point there were as many as 50 men in Brockley from the small village of Carisolo (in the Rendena valley in Trentino), which at the beginning of the new millennium had only 500 inhabitants. These men met (and those who remained at the time of our interviews still do) at the Wickham Arms, playing cards and talking about their village. Some Trentini became economically successful and some male offspring continued the family businesses, but overall the offspring maintained close-knit family and village-based networks while at the same time interacting much more than the previous group had done with British people and institutions (mainly through work and education).

With competition and success, knife-grinding Trentino families moved both to the south and north of the city. Although few of our interviewees lived in the original areas of settlement, several said that they had an Italian neighbour. Personal networks could be an explanation for this pattern. Rosa, for example, explained that she heard of the sale of the house that became her home from an Italian woman in church, and on deciding to buy the house was happy to know about her next-door neighbours.

There is also a more recent flow of Italians who have settled in Britain. They were comprised mainly of professionals and students, were highly heterogeneous, and scattered throughout London. In the main, the professionals were relocated to London by their companies or government institutions, but there was also a growing number of individuals who came in search of better employment opportunities. Many who came to study stayed on and sometimes married partners from outside their immediate communities; some have no links with the Italian communities. However, their links remain very strong with Italy and with their families at home.

As we will see in later chapters, Italian migrants harboured fears about their children marrying into non-Italian families and communities, partly because migrants wanted to return with their families intact. Second, while Italians in Britain shared many characteristics, there were also differences – for example, men generally wished to return to their homelands, while women wanted to stay so that they could be close to their children and grandchildren. This gender division around feelings and commitments was also common with the interviewees in Caribbean communities. Third, there was a tension between permanent settlement and return; again, this was a common feature in both sets of communities. For example, many Italians expressed a sense of being doubly excluded. While they felt that they were not fully socially and culturally integrated into British society, they were also no longer part of their villages of origin. Many said that they ended up complaining in both places – they would often defend 'Italian' ways in Britain, and 'English' ways in Italy. The situation was much the same for most Caribbeans.

Friendship bonds and social networks

The locations in which migrants settled and formed new communities strongly influenced the type of networks they and their offspring developed. Both Caribbean and Italian migrants tended to network and socialize with kin and others from the same village, town or parish. They also established friendships with people who had similar ethnic, racial and social class backgrounds whom they met at work, community associations, and places of worship. Not surprisingly, they tended to be more suspicious of people outside these circles, and thereby conformed to what is widely known about many migrant communities. Friendships, however, beyond the family, was a key resource for migrants, as Margherita, offspring of Italian migrants, observed:

> my parent's generation, they have good, strong, friendships which replicates a sense of family, given that we don't have any direct family. They are really good to each other and they share things and make wine together and cook together and bring presents to each other when they visit and they have a strong sense of friendship which for that generation is I think very important ... to give them a sense of continuity and familiarity.
>
> (Margherita, interview location: Aylesbury, April 2004)

Margherita's family were members of a tightly knit Italian community in Aylesbury, but even in London, where Italians are not geographically concentrated, elderly people of Italian origin seemed to have strong friendship networks based largely, although not exclusively, on their shared ethnicity. But while they met most of their friends through church or voluntary activities in associations and other groups, the church and the neighbourhood stood out as important places where some migrants extended their friendship networks into other ethnic groups.

The picture appeared less clear-cut for their children and later generations. Of course, friendship networks remained very important but the pattern was more complex compared with those of their immigrant parents. For British Italians, a shared ethnic background and similar lived experiences appeared to be the most important factors shaping some of their closest friendship networks. Giorgina, an offspring of Italian migrants, socialized with a mixture of people across diverse ethnic groups, but at the time of our interview most of her friends were from Italian backgrounds; she made a point of stressing that these friends were British-Italian, thereby indicating her awareness of the differences between this category and Italians from Italy as well as her distance from the latter. She reflected on the sadness of loosing close ties or bonds with the people from her parents' valley in Italy, when she said that

> the mentality of us that have grown up in London, that have worked hard, we know what it is to … those in Italy now who have got what they've got … now they tend to be a bit above themselves and they see us come to Carisolo, when I go I feel I'm the same person, I see my friends now in the street and I feel like giving them a hug and catching up as if they're as they were but they're not. Something's happened; they couldn't care less whether I went to see them.
>
> (Giorgina, interview location: London, January 2004)

Pia, on the other hand, who was born in Italy and lived in London for more than 40 years, was able to develop a rich network of Italian and non-Italian friends in London, but at the same time also managed to maintain her friendly relationships in Italy. She told us that she had

> at least I would say maybe about 10 [friends in Italy] which I see them three or four times a year and maybe 20 of which I see maybe once a year. … That's why I never really felt that I was … how can I say it? … that I was a foreigner here. From day one that I arrived here I have always gone back to Italy two or three times a year. So when you don't really cut yourself away from there, you feel 'All right you're a little bit far away from there' but you know, you still know what's going on and then when I used to be there we used to do things together.
>
> (Pia, interview location: London, March 2004)

Many respondents reported having had mixed friendship networks in the past but when asked about their present best friends many said they were Italians. For others, however, present best friends were not necessarily Italians but people who had similar experiences, such as the children of other immigrants. For Margherita this included individuals with shared sexual identities, such as her gay friends.

Similarly to our Caribbean respondents as we shall see below, offspring of Italian migrants reflected on their childhood and schooling years and the ways in which this informed their friendship relationships. They recalled that whilst they had a variety of friends from across a number of ethnic backgrounds in school, their parents did not allow them to invite these friends home. As a consequence, some kept secret friendships at school, whereas others preferred to socialize mainly with other Italian children or immigrant children who had similar restrictions placed on them by their parents, and were therefore able to understand the situation. One respondent, Claudia, remembered how she would socialize with young Italian people around the Italian church in south London, through social and sporting events such as the Sunday disco and football matches.

There were others, however, who found it difficult to fit into these ethnic-specific, homogeneous, networks and groups. For example, Claudia felt that she

> was different to them, like my brothers, my brothers were hippies, long hair, and these Italians with their clean suits and nice short hair and we smoked and real smoked and they knew that we, I wasn't ladylike let's say, I was in jeans, flares, clogs, I was different.
>
> (Claudia, interview location: London, March 2004)

Margherita had a strong Italian friendship network when she was young but as she grew older she felt that her friends' lack of ambition and conformity to the values of the Italian community were holding her back. When she started university Margherita established a friendship with an Italian woman of similar ethnic background, but the defining factor in their friendship was that her friend shared the same aspirations and ambitions in life. She told us that she

> met this ... one of my closest friends now ... on the same course and I'd never met an Italian girl like me before. She's older than me and comes from Peterborough but she had the same experience as me and I'd never met anyone like that. I thought I was a freak and I was very unconventional within the Italian community. So I met her and she had the same background as me and it was like, such a ... I think my life would have been very different if I had 20 friends like that when I was growing up. Part of my identity was formed through being different to the other ... not being like English people but not being like Italian people either.
>
> (Margherita, interview location: Aylesbury, April 2004)

With regards to the children of the Italian offspring, friendship choices appeared to have been different again when compared with those of their parents and their immigrant grandparents. This is especially true for those children living in large cities such as London. Their networks of friends seemed to be ethnically mixed and less influenced by their parents or ethnic group identity and membership, as the interview with Carolina suggested:

Q: What's the ethnic background of your friends?
A: Everything. Some Muslim ... in Italy where I go it's just Italian people and that's it! No Black people, no Chinese ... just all Italian people but in England or in London I have white and black friends, a few Italian friends, two Chinese friends, a Japanese friend ... a bit of everything really ... In my group there is two Muslims, a few English, Irish, some not even religious – atheists kind of thing – not even mainly English in my group! Mainly Irish the people I know ... half-Irish and half-English or half-Irish and half-Scottish! No real pure English

people in my group. Not one kid who is pure English and they all have a bit of something in them. They are all mixed.

(Carolina, interview location: London, May 2004)

In our interviews, the offspring of Caribbean migrants raised issues of how community and neighbourhood ties acted as an important social resource in developing friendship networks. These young people had high expectations of their close friends and they had strongly invested in the relationships they shared. The themes of reciprocal exchanges, trust, equality, honesty, uncritical support, loyalty, mutual understanding and 'being there' for each other occurred repeatedly in the young people's accounts of friendship. In London, Sharon told us about her

friend Marcel. I know that if something bugs me and I tell her, that it will go no further, because she'll just keep that confidence. We've got that understanding that we don't need to say, 'Do not tell anyone'; it's just taken as read. It's like an unspoken rule type of thing.

(Sharon, interview location: London, December 2003)

Migrants' offspring and their children whom we interviewed valued the stability and durability of their friendships and spoke about the ways that friends complemented specific aspects of personality. Carol's bubbling testimony of friendship revealed deep trust and confidence, when she confidently told us that

it works with my best friends because we're so different. You've got Emma, who's, like, the goody goody and you've got me who's kind of like in between, then you've got Clare who's really naughty. And I find we kind of gel off each other in that sense. They're the type of friends who are constant, and who wouldn't just be [there] at the good times.

(Carol, interview location: Nottingham, April 2004)

In many accounts the young people expressed a generalized view of same-ethnic friendships framed around trust, support and reciprocal bonds. However, in both explicit and implicit terms they also identified how shared ethnic and racial bonds provided the context for these reciprocal trust relationships. These strong bonding ties established through a shared ethnic identity encouraged affinity, familiarity and a sense of empathy between young people and their same-ethnic friends, as Patrice told us

Ciara and Missy are my only two friends who are fully Jamaican. Like both parents come from Jamaica, and that's why we have a lot in common. The conversations I have with Ciara and Missy I couldn't have with my other friends. We talk about the kind of food we're eating. Ciara may say 'What are you having in your soup?' I'll know she's talking about dinner on Saturday because we both know that Saturday is soup day. And because we share same background our conversations are deeper, we talk about our family here [in the UK] and Jamaica.

(Patrice, interview location: London, October 2003)

The Caribbean young people's experiences of school indicate that there were a number of factors that facilitated the development of same-ethnic friendships when moving to secondary school. The transition from primary to secondary school usually occurs when children are 11 years old and they are entering the adolescent phase of the life-course. Adolescence is a crucial time for children to begin to explore issues of identity, separate from that of their family and parents (Morrow 1999). For Caribbean children and adolescents who live in a white society, part of this identity-making is articulated in ethnic-racial terms. This involves a process of race awareness, the development of a racial self and sensitivity to racial difference. Many Caribbean offspring remarked that it was during their adolescent years that for the first time they felt different or excluded from white school friends and they had experienced direct (or open) racial discrimination. Consequently, when they started secondary school they tended racially to identify with other black children. These friendship networks also acted as a protective buffer and support mechanism in the face of real (or perceived) instances of racial discrimination by other children and teachers. Moving to secondary school meant moving out of their local neighbourhoods into a wider social and physical space, which gave them the chance to meet a wider network of black children from neighbouring communities. Patrice's recollections of her friends during her transition from primary to secondary school illustrate this point:

At primary school, all my friends were black and two of them were white. We [friends] all applied for [the same school] but I was the only one to get in. It was a good school and the majority of children that go there are white and middle-class. It was in a good area, not our area, but further out from where I lived. So I had to leave all my friends, and I had to make new friends. My main friends in secondary school were black because we had to stick together because they weren't many black girls in that school. They used to say we were a gang because we all hung around together and we were all black, whereas the majority of school was white. We used to get told off and always getting into trouble with the teachers, saying we was 'too loud' and we had 'too much attitude' but we were just sticking up for ourselves. Besides we were good at our work, I left with 10 GCSEs with four of them A* [grades] and my friends also got loads of GCSEs too so they [teachers] really couldn't tell us anything because we did get on with our work but they [teachers] just didn't like us, they [teachers] couldn't relate to us.

(Patrice, interview location: London, October 2003)

It is also useful to consider how aspects of the school curriculum and the practice of streaming children according to academic ability could contribute to the salience of same-ethnic friendship networks in multi-ethnic secondary school. As children's school friendship choices are mostly established with children in the same year group and classes, this creates a potential situation whereby Caribbean children, disproportionately concentrated in lower academic streams, are choosing other same-ethnic friends who are also located within these groups. Similarly, the minority of students of Caribbean backgrounds in the higher academic stream may band together for support and protection.

By and large it was the young people who attended comprehensive schools in working-class and multi-cultural communities who had a greater tendency to develop same-ethnic friendships. In contrast, young people who moved from predominantly white primary schools to predominantly white secondary schools in affluent areas tended to have friends from different ethnic groups. Those young people who attended private sector secondary schools also had greater tendency to develop multi-racial social networks of friends. Sometimes these young people later developed a racialized consciousness, for example, at university or the workplace, or they utilized other social resources within their social networks, such as transnational family and kinship relationships, to construct new or revised ethnic identities.

Two of our Caribbean respondents, Justin and Anthony, attended private schools and they discussed these experiences during our interviews. Justin, who was 16-years-old was still at school and Anthony, who was 20-years-old had left school. Both Justin and Anthony lived in a professional two-parents middle-class home, in affluent outer London suburbs. In Justin's case, only a handful of black (mainly African) children attended his school, and his friends came from diverse racial and ethnic backgrounds. On the advice and guidance of his parents Justin strategically selected his friends on the basis of developing future relationships and contacts that could help him later in life. The additional economic resources available to him at school also created greater opportunities to participate in extra-curricular activity, which promoted inter-ethnic mixing. So, for example, Justin was a keen sportsman and represented his school in cricket, football, hockey, rugby and swimming. He also attended the school's annual skiing trips to Austria where he socialized within a racially diverse network. The bonding factor in Justin's friendship networks was shared socio-economic status. In turn, Justin was able to use these bonds to make a bridge across ethnic groups.

Anthony's experiences provide a different perspective concerning inter-ethnic friendship networks established in a privately funded predominantly white secondary school. Anthony reflected that his parents had a race-conscious approach to bringing up children and this was instrumental in his developing race awareness and an ethnic identity at a very young age. In addition, when Anthony was a small child, his father accepted a senior government post in Guyana and the entire family relocated. He thus completed his formative education in Guyana. When his family returned to the UK in the mid-1990s he attended a secondary school where he was the only black child in his year group. Anthony felt that his experiences of living in the Caribbean during his formative years, alongside his parents' attitudes, made him very aware of his ethnic-racial identity from a young age. These factors provided him with the confidence to develop multi-racial networks of friends whilst at the same time being embedded in his own racial and ethnic identities.

The social networks that parents establish or are members of also influenced the type of identity and networks children developed. Parents, who were strongly involved in ethnic organizations such as black supplementary schools and other ethnic-specific events, were more likely to instil in their children a strong sense of ethnic and racial identities. Likewise, middle-class parents were more likely to have social networks that transcended neighbourhood boundaries and they were able to more successfully use these social networks to provide social contacts and guidance to their children compared with working-class and low-income parents. Interestingly, some of these Caribbean parents saw themselves in a dilemma over ensuring that their children did not grow up in environments and neighbourhoods that were 'too ethnic' or 'too black' and assuming negative values with black youth cultural identity and a concern about the psychological effects of their children loosing their cultural roots as a result of having exclusively white and English friendship networks and neighbourhoods. This was not an option or a concern for working-class parents who tended to live in multi-ethnic areas.

Higher education also played a crucial role in consolidating the young people's networks along racial and ethnic lines. As discussed elsewhere, it was noticeable that many young people chose to attend local universities in black and urban areas where other black students also attended, instead of institutions that may have been better resourced (and may have provided them with better opportunities) where there were limited numbers of black students. They tended to take courses where there were a relatively high numbers of black students and which provided a greater degree of success and future career opportunities, suggesting that they thought in strategic terms about their educational and career choices. As Angela in Birmingham told us

> I wasn't really sure what social work was but I know that they had plenty of black people on the course and you see that other black people have careers in that area. I really wanted to do the librarian course at [university] but some subjects, you rarely find black people working in that area. Whilst in areas like social work and social housing there's more opportunities and you have a fair chance of completing and getting a good job at the end.
>
> (Angela, interview location: Birmingham, December 2003)

The few young people who did venture out to institutions in largely mono-ethnic provincial areas found that they often felt isolated and alienated from their white peers and one strategy to cope with the situation was to actively seek out friendships with other black and minority ethnic students who they could rely on for support. For Emma, therefore, part

> of the process of us three getting together was when we was in college, we kind of got forced to be just friends, but it kind of lasted. We were the only black girls on the course, the rest were white [girls] and no one wanted to work with us, so we did what we had to do and everyone was like 'we're not talking to them'. We became really close friends because of all the problems we were

having in class and stuff, and so we all supported each other to get each other through the course because we were all going through the same thing.

(Emma, interview location: London, April 2005)

University life created the space, opportunity and networking possibilities for black students to meet and socialize with other black students and further explore issues of ethnic and racial identities through their participation in ethnic-specific events. These experiences in the university setting created friendship networks for the young people, some of which survived after graduation. In the work setting, same-ethnic friendships were also likely to develop. Caribbean people tend to be concentrated and sometimes over-represented in some employment sectors, while under-represented in others (Modood *et al.* 1997; Strategy Unit 2003). This commonality of experience or a perception tends to promote greater ethnic solidarity.

Conclusion

In this part of our discussion, we have pointed to aspects of generational change in friendship patterns for migrants, offspring and their children. Whilst the migrants' friendship networks tend to be singularly influenced by close-knit and ethnic-specific communities, generally the picture is less clear-cut for their offspring and later generations. For these groups a range of factors including racio-ethnic identities, educational and schooling experience, participation in ethnic association, community and recreational activities, combine with place of settlement to inform their friendship patterns and networks.

6 Families, needs and caring practices

Introduction

It is generally assumed that migration undermines reciprocal family relationships, particularly with regard to providing care for needy members. However, as we indicated in an earlier chapter, the provision of care for family and kinship members across national boundaries is a key factor that maintains transnational families. The care with which we are concerned is not that which migrants provide for others, but that which they provide for themselves and family members in different parts of the world, and in this chapter we focus on two important aspects. We describe these caring activities as *caring about* each other, and *caring for* each other in order to highlight activities which may be understood as points along a continuum rather than sharp distinctions of kinds of care or caring. Thus, *caring about* and *caring for* activities include a diverse range of reciprocal and practical caring work performed by members of families dispersed across geographical spaces. This chapter explores these aspects of transnational care, but it is necessary first to situate our discussion within a more general context.

Understanding care and support in minority ethnic families

The rich body of literature on the feminist ethic of care has influenced our analysis of care and support in ethnic minority families and has helped us move beyond conventional understandings of care as one-directional and originating from a single source, flowing from a care-giver (the 'haves') to a care-receiver (the 'haves not') (Sevenhuijsen 2000; Ackers and Stalford 2004). In social policy terms, this viewpoint is supported by a discourse of kinship care that focuses on those people who are dependent and in need of financial and personal care. For example, in the field of health and social care, care services primarily focus on particular stages of the life course – babies and young children, the elderly and the infirm, the disabled and relatively poor, and the socio-economically disadvantaged (Edwards *et al.* 1999; Williams 2005). Related to this dependency model of care is the idea that as individuals become more upwardly mobile and independent, they regard themselves as being less in need of care and support, thereby strengthening a sense of the autonomous individual (Beck 1992). The phenomenon of individualism has been extensively discussed in relation to the changing nature of social and moral ties that bind individuals and family networks together (see, Beck and Gernsheim 2002; McRae 1997; Irwin 1999). In positive terms, it has been argued that individualism gives rise to diverse family arrangements and more personal autonomy, but it has also given rise to the increasing fragmentation and dispersal of families, and thereby making it necessary for families to be dependent on public provision. While this view cannot be entirely dismissed, it is also important to acknowledge the care provided by family members themselves for each other.

We therefore want to challenge or modify the dependency model of care where new communities in Britain are concerned on two grounds. First, our data illustrates that Caribbean and Italian families have caring relationships that are reciprocal and multi-directional. Family members are active in both giving and receiving care provision, irrespective of their social and economic status. We identified three ways in which reciprocal relationships work in families:

- inter-generationally (between parents and children, grand-parents and grand-children, uncles and aunts and nephews, and so on.)
- intra-generationally (between siblings, cousins)
- transnationally (when reciprocity operates among family members across geographical boundaries).

Secondly, our findings indicate that there is little evidence to suggest that family members are less involved in caring relationships as a result of growing individualism. For example, while individualism is a dominant aspect of Caribbean society and culture, and there exists greater autonomy for individuals to choose their lifestyles, family forms and living arrangements (Goulbourne 2002), family connections and responsibilities are maintained. They undertake collective and individual responsibility for care within this individualized framework because the individualized self is understood as relational and situational to others within their networks. In contrast, in Italian and southern European families, despite increased diversity in living arrangements, the individual is still understood to be less autonomous and more interwoven into the family. Italian families have been going through structural changes, which include the decline of the extended family. Whilst extended households are no longer as common in southern Europe as they were, family members continue to live close to one another, maintaining important economic and emotional links. What strikes many observers of Italian society is the centrality of the family, and their apparent stability and cohesion (Finch 1989a).

As one would expect, there are cultural differences in the ways in which the relationships between the individual and the family are articulated in the two communities. In general terms, while it may be said that Caribbeans are likely to have a specifically negotiated, situational or relational relationship with family and kin members, Italians are more tightly ascriptively connected or grounded. A degree of commonality exists, however, in the ways in which individuals in these communities are embedded in webs of personal relationships and utilize social capital as a resource (Griffiths 1995). Care provision is a case in point. It represents an important family and social resource for connecting and relating to other family

members. This understanding of caring networks that views the individual as relational, interconnected and embedded in their personal relationships chimes with
much feminist scholarship where it is recognized that care is a daily process of
social action framing interactions (Finch 1989b; Fisher and Tronto 1990; Thorne
and Yalom 1992; Griffiths 1995; Clement 1996; Mackenzie and Stoljar 2000;
Sevenhuijsen 2000).

It is for this reason that we have adopted the feminist distinction between caring
about and caring for (Finch and Groves 1983; Fisher and Tronto 1990; Ackers and
Stalford 2004). We understand caring about to encompass contact and emotional
support connected to sociability, advice, comfort and self-validation. Examples of
caring about activities include communication by telephone, letters, emails, visits,
participation in family decision-making and financing the purchase of care (Di
Leonardo 1992). We understand caring for to refer to concrete, 'hands-on' care-
giving on a personal level (Finch and Groves 1983; Ackers and Stalford 2004).

There is a moral dimension to the understanding of caring about and caring for
in kin relationships in family and kinship networks. Finch and Mason (1993) cham-
pions the concept of 'kinship morality' to suggest that a set of moral discourses
informs our behaviour towards kin members. Similarly, Williams (2005: 55) suggests that people negotiate their relationship within these moral guidelines and they
act as moral agents involved in negotiating 'the proper thing to do' in and through
their commitments to others. These caring commitments, Williams argues, 'cross
the boundaries of blood, marriage, residence, culture and country' (ibid.).

Finally, it must be noted that issues of identity, belonging and loyalty to the family in different geographical locations are of vital importance when considering the
caring practices of transnational families. The early literature on transnationalism
had interpreted migrants' need to keep up links and networks with their country
of origin as a sign of their marginalization and precarious position in their countries of settlement (Glick-Schiller *et al.* 1992). While this is partly the case, our
evidence suggests that there is a far greater compulsion that motivates continuing
transnational links through care, and this compulsion is a combination of the sense
of responsibility and obligation as well as the felt needs for identity and belongingness irrespective of location, space and frequency of physical togetherness.

In the remainder of this chapter, we consider the two dimensions of care – caring about, and caring for – as ways of exploring the daily caring practices of our
respondents. Their accounts also serve to highlight differences according to racial
and ethnic, gender, generational, territorial and other identities that define these
transnational families.

Caring about in minority ethnic families

Caring about family members and the *kin work* to which it gives rise assume a
crucial relevance for geographically dispersed families in the context of international migration. The very existence of transnational families does, in fact, rest
on kin ties being kept alive over great distances and prolonged separations, as we
explained in the first part of this book. Goulbourne and Chamberlain (2001: 42), in

their study of transnational Caribbean families, found that 'geographical distance
is no barrier to being a "close" family and respondents in their study stressed the
importance of transnational links in maintaining the "tightness" of the emotional
bonds, and the level of "trust" expected and experienced between family members'.
Goulbourne (2002: 196) returns to this theme in a later study where he highlights
that transnational care between family members reinforces 'continuity and bonding
across distance'. This is especially important when generational differences and
cultural divides mark the potential to produce distance between family members.
For a number of minority ethnic families in the UK, migration represents the social
context in which much of the caring work and responsibility takes places within
family networks (Peach 1991; Ahmed 1993; Ahmed and Atkin 1996; Goulbourne
and Solomos 2003). Migration creates and maintains reciprocal caring relationships
between those family members left behind and those who migrated elsewhere in
search of better opportunities. These transnational caring networks reinforce a
sense of cultural or ethnic belongingness amongst participating members.

Multi-directional 'caring about' practices, obligations and responsibilities
operated within family networks in a number of ways. Caring about tasks and
responsibilities ranged from providing small favours to family members such
as money loans, telephoning family members and giving advice, support, or just
merely 'checking in' about the welfare of a family member. Caring about each
other included organizing regular family meals with married children and their
new families; family celebrations such as birthdays, Christmas and Easter; regular
visits 'back home' to the Caribbean and Italy; hosting kin members in the UK, and
gift-giving, as Werbner also found amongst Pakistanis in Britain (Werbner 2002).
We found that family members devote considerable time and energies to these
tasks, despite geographical distances and time differences.

These observations led us to think of some of these exchanges and relationships
as a form of *cultural remittance* and we expect this notion to help us advance our
understanding of *caring about* relationships. Cultural remittance represents people's emotional attachments and the ways in which migrants abroad utilize their
family links to maintain cultural connections to their place of origin (Burman
2002). Other forms of cultural remittance include owning and building property
'back home', the celebration of cultural rituals and national events in the new
country of residence and keeping abreast of national news 'back home' through
the Internet and newspapers. Cultural remittance reinforces ethnic identity and is
viewed as a sign of the continued commitment to the kinship group left behind
and a commitment to keeping these members together. The most common type of
'kin-keeping' or keeping kinship ties alive occurred between siblings, parents and
children, and grandparents and grandchildren.

The commitment to keeping the family together was discussed by many of our
respondents. Lucille, one of our Caribbean respondents in London, strongly illustrates this point. She stated that:

> there's always a lot of phoning going on to see how everyone is doing. ...
> You know when mum went back to Barbados about 15 years now, it would

be so easy for us to drift apart, so when she left we had to take stock ... and say 'right, mum's not here now, so it's down to us to keep it together, we're going to put the effort into making time for each other doesn't matter how busy, families got to come first', so we try and meet at one of ours [brothers and sisters], all cousins playing with each other, we take it in turns ... to cook Sunday dinner. ... I'm not saying that we've not had our differences and disputes, that normal in any family but we make time for each other, you've got to put those differences aside don't you? ... because at the end of the day family's all you got isn't it?

(Lucille, interview location: London, March, 2004)

Spending time together, visiting each other and having family dinners are ways of keeping families together that are available only to those kin members who live in close proximity. When distance is a problem, the easiest and most frequent way in which *caring about* is expressed by family members is by telephone calls for migrants and, increasingly, particularly by their offspring, the Internet; these means of communication enable members to keep in contact with their cousins and other relatives who are of the same generation. Through these means families feel that they are kept together; they update scattered members about what is going on in each other's lives; and they provide emotional support. Crucially, they direct and organize needed hands-on care from family members.

Thus, for a while Carmela spoke daily on the phone to her brother in Switzerland and their mother in Italy, and these siblings were very conscious of their responsibility for their mother at a distance. Another way in which families maintain a sense of connection across distance and show their commitment towards each other is through 'gift-giving'. Carmela terms this 'signs of love', and explains, thus

I always send something to my mum for her birthday, because she's old, I send her a jumper, a nightgown, anything. Mum is very happy when she get them, not because she needs them, because she has her pension, but because it's a sign of love.

(Carmela, interview location: Peterborough, March 2004)

The activities of sending and receiving food items have a similar symbolic relevance centring on caring for and about each other. In spite of the increased availability of such items in the markets in many parts of Britain, the direct supply of food from relatives in Italy and the Caribbean appear to be expected and much appreciated. This may be because such items remind individuals of close ones, particular places and precious memories.

Perhaps the single most important way in which kin connections are kept across the generations is through the frequency of visits 'home' (Baldassar 2001). This event is very important for renewing and reaffirming cultural identity for migrants, their immediate offspring and grandchildren. Such visits are strongly linked to the presence of family members at the point of original departure. Italians and their offspring use these visits 'home' to invest in properties, looked after by their family or kinship members, and used when visiting on holidays. The same is true to one degree or another for some Caribbeans, although their properties may also be rented, and while visiting they might stay with relatives and friends. The importance of such investments 'back home' will be returned to in the chapter on the phenomenon of 'return'. However, it is worth noting here how such investments feature in the preparation for return:

Q: My goodness, this is a huge house! Just the two of you live here?
A: Yes, but we built it big because when we retired it was our dream to come back home so we started making plans early so that everything in place to start building before we retired. It was our life ambition to have a big house, with lots of space … in England we're cooped up in these small pokey houses and there's no space …. And after living like that in England for nearly 40 years it was enough. This place isn't just for us you know, the kids are always coming with the grandchildren, we wanted them to feel comfortable and there's plenty of space for them and when we go [die], it's left for them so its an investment.
(Pauline, interview location: Guyana, July 2004)

With regards to the migrants' offspring, we found that several of them felt that keeping links with their parents' country of origin was important. In some cases their educational and career choices were influenced by this 'need' to spend time in their respective territories. Marta's statement demonstrates this point when she stressed that

I've worked on and off, nothing fantastic, waitressing, in the market, waitressing, a lot of waitressing, that sort of stuff, I'm not a big …, I wasn't a career woman, I used to work for 11 months and then go to Italy for a month, 'cos you could do that then, and then come back and get another job, years ago you could do that, … I used to go to Italy, all the friends are up there, all the cousins are up there for the holidays, spend all staying out hanging about.
(Marta, interview location: London, November 2003)

Young people of Caribbean origin also identified the emotional and psychological support they felt they received from these visits 'home'. In their view, this allowed them to develop a positive sense of well-being and sense of belonging, which counteracted their felt sense of racial discrimination, inequality and exclusion in Britain.

Italian migrants' children also valued the visits 'home' as an important resource in reinforcing their felt ethnic identity. However, in contrast to young people of Caribbean backgrounds, young people of Italian heritage balanced the positive value they gained from these trips with the obligation they felt in undertaking the visits, the pain and anxiety caused by the anticipation of separation, and the unsettlement provoked by the experience of the visit.

These attitudes by the Caribbean and Italians offspring can be best explained by the distance and proximity of these family visits 'home'. With the exception of a few respondents who made annual visits 'home', the majority of Caribbean offspring made infrequent visits on a biannual or longer basis. In many instances their parents had returned and settled in an area where they did not have family roots or kinship ties. Therefore, whilst they valued their strong family bonds in the Caribbean, they were often less attached than those of Italian heritage to places of family origins. Our British-Caribbean were, therefore, less likely than our Italian respondents to experience anxiety and guilt about obligations when they visited their immigrant parents' 'home'.

'Caring for' in minority ethnic families

Our interviewees' accounts of daily activities and family relationships provided a wealth and a range of multi-directional examples of transnational *caring for* provisions between family members. The most commonly cited included care between siblings; between grandparents and grandchildren; parents and children; and between more fortunate and less fortunate family members. These 'caring for' practices included domestic help such as childcare and financial assistance such as remittances. Sometimes their caring exchanges reflected specific and regular tasks and responsibilities, but more often than not care took the form of less defined everyday activities that were not generally thought of as care provision. This reluctance to describe what they did as care provision suggests that many family members saw such care as part of everyday life. They regarded themselves as fulfilling responsibilities and obligations to the family. Often these reciprocal exchanges were immediate and concurrent (exchanging caring services at the same time); sometimes these provisions were given at different times and stages in a person's life course – situations in which individuals provide care in the present in expectation of future reciprocal care for themselves. In the remainder of this section we use inter-generational care and sibling care to illustrate our general point about practices of caring for each other.

It has long been recognized in Caribbean family studies that grandparents and other senior family members care for dependent children left behind by parents who migrated (see, for example, Brodber 1974; Senior 1991; Fog Olwig 1993; Russell-Browne *et al.* 1997; Reynolds 2005). A large number of mothers who migrated were from low-income socio-economic groups, they often did not have the economic means to take their children with them, and in any event most had the intention of returning within a relatively short time. In these circumstances, many mothers and family members thought that the child's best interest was to stay behind and be cared for by relatives. Latoya, from Jamaica, related to us how she moved between her father's and her grandmother's homes, before she joined her mother in London

> [she] came here [UK], and then she came back to Jamaica, and then she left again, for a while, before she send for us. So I was living there with my dad and his girlfriend, but we didn't get on. We used to argue all the time because she [girlfriend] was jealous that I was close to my dad, so my grandmother

said 'bring her come, mek me care her'. So I lived there with my granny and it was nice, I lived there with my auntie and cousins in a big house in Vineyard Town [Kingston]. When I was 15 my mum just called and said to me, 'Oh, I'm going to send for you guys', like me and my sister, so I was just looking forward to come here and starting living a new life with her.

(Latoya, interview location: London, February 2004)

Throughout the period of migration across the Atlantic and to North America from the 1950s, grandparents have provided similar care. Indeed, four or more decades after mass migration to Britain, parents who had now become grandparents themselves participated in caring for grandchildren. The relative ease and affordability of air travel facilitated regular and frequent visits in both directions across the Atlantic by grandparents as care-givers. Plaza (2000) has aptly described this as the 'flying grandmother' phenomenon (see also, Goulbourne and Chamberlain 2001).

There have also been cases when grandchildren visited grandparents in the Caribbean during school holidays in Britain, and in this way grandparents continued to provide childcare. This arrangement provided Daniel with cherished memories with his grandparents and cousins in Jamaica:

Q: How often did you go to Jamaica?

A: Every summer she [mum] sent me to stay with grandparents and cousins in JA until I was about fifteen. Every summer my grandmother look after me

Q: And what things did you do there?

A: Me and my cousins we'd pick oranges and ackee off the tree with her (grandmother), and we helped her prepare the food and stuff. And the kids in Jamaica are trained with more manners and respect for olders .... Every Saturday morning, I'd have to get up early and go to the market, with my gran, shopping. She watched all the soaps [tv soap operas] ... it was my job to set the recorder, I taught her how to use it because she didn't know how to work the video-recorder.

(Daniel, interview location: Manchester, November 2003)

Daniel's recollection highlights how inter-generational learning and mutual exchange of knowledge between grandparent and grandchild may be an important facet of care provision. In the process Daniel's grandmother also transmitted cultural norms and social values (for example, social manners and etiquette) and educated him about life in Jamaica. From Daniel's perspective, in turn, he was able to teach his grandmother new skills, such as setting the video recorder to record her favourite TV programmes. Other young people in our study identified their role and responsibility towards elderly family members and helping them to acquire new skills and building confidence in using new technology, such as the Internet, CD/DVD players and digital cameras, which grandchildren would sometimes provide. Such inter-generational learning is not generally regarded as care provision, but these interactions can help to maintain emotional bonds and strengthen family connections even where families live most of the time in different countries.

Families of Italian heritage in Britain articulate a similar narrative of their experiences. Migrant women had a heavy burden when they first arrived. They worked full time in factories and had sole responsibility for the home, their husbands and their children, and of course they were initially cut off from the support provided by other family members. Although husbands and friends played a bigger role than they would have done in Italy, nonetheless the women carried the main burden for the family's welfare. Not unlike their Caribbean counterparts, some women became 'transnational mothers' and also sent their children to school in Italy. This particularly occurred when there was a plan for the family to return permanently to Italy. As the return was not always achieved, children and young people often had to re-adapt to life in Britain, after spending several years away from the country and their immediate family.

Children of Italian migrants had quickly to learn to look after themselves as well as carry out important tasks for their parents, such as conducting translations and filling in forms. Francesco told us that

> we started integrating speaking English and then obviously if they [parents] ever needed to go anywhere we would always have to go with them .... If my parents had to go to a doctor or to the hospital or to do anything and sometimes even to the shops ... I would have to go with them and interpret what was going on.
>
> (Francesco, interview location: Bedford, March 2004)

Italian migrant women, who missed out looking after their children when they were young due to their work commitments, later became heavily involved with their grandchildren. Grandfathers also played a significant, although different, role. Some grandparents even changed their retirement plans in order to fulfil what they regarded as their responsibility. Franco described his new role as carer of his grandchild thus:

> We now have another kid at the age of 50, but he gives us lots back so it is worth living like this for a few years. But he changed our life really. ... In the sense that we are not free anymore, that's all ... I thought it was a bit hard because we had just started one or two years before to go on holiday two or three times per year and then all of a sudden we found ourselves that we couldn't do that anymore. Before we couldn't do it because we couldn't afford it, now that we can afford it we can't do it. It's not the time but the freedom we should have, but having said that the boy gives us a lot of satisfaction which I wouldn't change with anything. ... I take him to the park, we spend time together at home, we spend time on holiday.
>
> (Franco, interview location: London, October 2003)

In case of their children's divorce, grandparents support can become especially crucial if they are called upon to provide housing, babysitting and financial support. Cristina's story illustrates these points, when she told us about her mother's support she said we'll live together and it was the best thing that could have happened to me and my children because I was able to go to work and so I could support them ... and I was able to afford all the classes ... the swimming and the clarinet and everything because I was with my mum and I didn't have to pay rent ... Italian ... it's the culture and I had security and if I ever wanted to go out in the evening I knew the children were at home.

(Cristina, interview location: London, November 2003)

There are also 'flying grandmothers' in Italian families, as in Rita's case; for sometime she travelled to Italy to her granddaughter every five or six weeks:

It's 11 years now that I am faithfully there every five or six weeks at the most. ... it's not something that I have to do, it's an enjoyment 'cos I really want to see her growing up and I want to enjoy her while I can ... I take her shopping and buy her whatever she needs and you know how we are? We like to spoil our grandchildren ... everything is pleasure and it's not because I have to.

(Rita, interview location: London, December 2003)

These examples of reciprocal caring exchanges in Italian and Caribbean families illustrate how grandparents are an important resource in terms of the emotional and financial support they provide. They also show how the grandparent–grandchild interaction is significant in maintaining kinship ties and family networks (see, for example, Gray 2005; Wolf 2004). In both cases, the grandparents acknowledged that they derived satisfaction and personal pleasure from looking after their grandchildren, but not all enjoyed babysitting. Some were unhappy that it was expected that they would provide free childcare for their grandchildren, and this sometimes became a source of tension in the family.

Care for the elderly was also done transnationally. In the Caribbean, elderly retired returnees often relied on family members in Britain for help and assistance, because public health facilities in the region are inadequate. The absence of universal health and social welfare may place pressing demands on family members at a distance across the Atlantic (see, Goulbourne 2002, ch. 7). Jocelyn's story is an example of this problem:

Mamma aunt suffers from sugars [diabetes] and pressure [hypertension] so I buy her medicine and see that she gets to the doctors to check for sugars and pressure. That's money for transport into town, money for the doctors and money for the medicine. It's stressful because there's time you think 'where am I going to find the money to pay the Doctor for the medicine this month and take care of mamma aunt' because it's so expensive. In England we're lucky you know ... you don't have to worry if you get sick, but over here [Guyana] everything is money. If you don't have money and you're sick, then it's your family you have to lean on to help out or you die, it stressful but what can you do? You have to pay.

(Jocelyn, interview location: Guyana, July 2004)

Italian migrants in Britain have also been preoccupied with their caring responsibility for ageing parents left in Italy. Often their care is devolved to other relatives still living in Italy. For middle-class professional migrants, there is the expectation that they will travel often to Italy so that they can continue to be fully involved in the care of ageing parents; this was part of Rita's experience.

> Well, I go about every five or six weeks. Usually if there is not a problem I just go for a long weekend. Like I go Wednesday and come back on the Monday, or Thursday and come back on the Monday. If there is a problem and he calls me then I'll go and I'll probably stay one week or 10 days or two weeks.
> (Rita, interview location: London, December 2003)

Ageing parents who lived in Britain was another problem that affected Italian families. Whilst adult children felt responsible for their parents, the children were sometimes concerned about how best to provide care. They were torn between the Italian ideal of having the elderly cared for in the home by family members and putting their parents in residential homes to be cared for by professional outsiders. The latter option often produced feelings of guilt about not living up to cultural values and norms concerning family care. Thus, Maria told us that

> my father went into a home but it was quite near us so we able to see him and he used to come home not every Sunday but quite a lot of Sundays, we'd go and get him and he'd come home for lunch ... then after my father died my mum was still living next door but about a year or two after that she became immobile, very confused, she became very lonely ... and after a while she went to live at Villa St Maria, it's not far from us ... but she needed full-time care, and she died five years ago ... I think most people whose parents go into homes ... it's a very guilty feeling that you have.
> (Maria, interview location: London, November 2003)

Although we have stressed the crucial role of families in providing care, the role of friendship networks and community organizations should not be overlooked. Whereas children help with transport, dealing with doctors and bureaucratic matters, sometimes it was friends who provided some day-to-day emotional support. At the age of 79 Salavatore and his wife enjoyed the support of their children, but they also had a variety of social networks outside the family. He had a very large friendship network and he was a member of various social clubs, some sponsored by the local council and targeting the large Italian population in Bedford. Moreover, the close-knit Italian communities in cities like Bedford and Peterborough provide important support for their ageing Italian immigrants. Francesca, of Italian ancestry and from Aylesbury, spoke positively about the community in Bedford:

> I think for that generation it's a positive thing ... my parent's generation, they have good strong friendships which replicates a sense of family, given that we don't have any direct family. They are really good to each other and they

share things and make wine together and cook together and bring presents to each other when they visit and they have a strong sense of friendship which for that generation is I think very important ... to give them a sense of continuity and familiarity.

(Francesca, interview location: London, March 2004)

Our second example of *caring for* is that between siblings. One of the main features of such care appeared to be its gender differentiation (see, Di Leonardo 1984; Mand 2002). In both studies, there were gender differences concerning the type of care people provide and the ways in which they expressed their caring commitments. Female kin were heavily involved in providing practical domestic caring work, childcare and contributing to 'kin-keeping' (Bornat *et al.* 1999; Williams 2005). Male siblings tended to involve themselves more with financial support, whilst female siblings identified childcare as their primary caring work in sibling relationships. Tamara reflected on how her uncle, who migrated from the Caribbean to Britain in the early 1960s, provided financial support to his younger brother and sisters and in so doing enabled them to move out of poverty in Jamaica during the 1970s. She recollected that her

parents were able to move up into middle-class because my uncle in London helped to educate his younger brothers and sisters. He worked as a bus driver for over 30 years, and would send money back. He also helped to put my five younger brothers and sisters through school, because we all went to good school in Kingston, but it was private school ... so that we all have a decent education, we've all got degrees and we're all doing professionals jobs .... People often forget that it's the working class who help to build middle class in Jamaica, it was down to my uncle that we became middle class.

(Marianna, interview location: Jamaica, June 2003)

Female siblings regularly participated in childcare for younger siblings and their siblings' children, nephews and nieces. Of Caribbean background, Makeba lived in London, and described a complex set of support and sibling dependence, when he said that

I'm always looking after my niece. I think she's the only person that I have to actually look after a lot – my brother's baby – and especially now, where he's split up with his girlfriend. He loves his child and everything, but he has to go out a lot and do things, he's a carpenter, and he does private jobs as well, and he always needs me, because my other brother, he's a footballer, and he's always out training, so there's no one really to help him out, and it's always me. And I don't mind anyway.

(Makeba, interview location: London, October 2003)

Females also tended to be family members who facilitated contact and maintained ties between geographically dispersed or estranged members; they were more likely to help maintain continuing relationship with ex-partners and their family members. Where there are cultural and generational differences females also played an active role in maintaining links. As noted, male kin were much more likely to provide financial assistance such as remittance to help pay for repairs, goods and other services such as paying for carers or helpers for family members in need. Speaking of her male siblings, Sophia recalled that

> They're always sending money back home, because they get a lot of letters, oh, like, 'It's hard out here, can you send us something?' But I think the time when they get a lot of those letters is when people know that they're coming to Jamaica, and then all the letters come in, with a long list of what people want them to buy.
>
> (Sophia, interview location: London, April 2004)

The 'caring for' provisions in transnational family networks therefore involves remittance of social resources (Reynolds and Zontini 2006; Thomas-Hope 2009), but it has been the economic dimension of remittance that has received greater attention in the literature. This is not surprising because the very existence of cross-national networks is often sustained through economic remittances (Carling 2002).

For example, remittances to the Caribbean region included the sending of consumer goods to family members and others (such as food and clothing) as well as money for maintaining family properties or for meeting educational or medical expenses (see, Millennium Development Report 2004). In general, financial remittances are widely regarded as having a positive contribution to families, households and local economies, and in many poor households remittance has been the primary source of family income (Vickerman 1999). However, such reliance on remittance can reduce a family members' ability independently to care for themselves and limit governments' commitment to welfare for their citizens (see, Conway 1993). Additionally, it has been suggested that economic remittances may be contributing to the decline of a work ethic by encouraging a dependency culture among the younger generations (Chevannes 1996). Economic remittances may therefore stifle local development because people spend what has been generated abroad on commodities from abroad.

Economic remittances are no longer such a significant aspect of Italian transnational family life, although such support used to be vitally important when Italy's economic situation was precarious. Much research in the 1970s and 1980s assessed the impact of remittances and return migration to Italy (see, King 1977), and the general conclusion was that remittances were primarily channelled to consumption and house building, thus scarcely benefiting the local communities. This is not the view of our interviewees, who feel that their role as emigrants was crucial for setting in motion the economic development of their countries. At present they feel bitter for having been forgotten in their 'home' country and for how things have turned out for them. They feel that often (at least in the north) those who had stayed behind were better off than those who had emigrated. As Franco told us,

> I don't know what I would do if I could go back in time. People who stayed
> behind are as well off now as those who left. I'm not sure … maybe I would
> do everything again, I'm happy how my family and work have turned out but
> there are other Italian emigrants who live a very hard life.
>
> (Franco, interview location: London, October 2003)

But although the economic need for remittances is no longer present, migrants
have not stopped transferring resources 'back home'. At the time of our interviews
this transfer took place mainly through the purchase or renovation of properties
and the sending of presents. Economic remittances have been transformed into
cultural remittances, aimed at keeping and strengthening emotional ties with the
places of origin. Cultural remittance represents another form of inter-generational
and transnational relationships migrants and their offspring participate in. As we
saw in Chapter 5, cultural remittance reflects people's emotional attachments
and represents the ways in which migrants abroad utilize their family links to
maintain cultural connections to their place of origin. Examples of cultural
remittance include owning and building property 'back home', the celebration
of cultural rituals and national events in the new country of residence and keeping abreast of national news 'back home' through the Internet and newspapers.
Cultural remittance reinforces ethnic identity in the country of settlement and
is viewed as a sign of the continued commitment to the kin left behind and
'kin-keeping'.

Social remittance is the third form of remittance by transnational kinship members, which is also present in our analysis. Social remittance is defined as 'the ideas,
behaviour, identities and social capital that flow from receiving to sending country
communities' (Levitt 1998: 926). In essence, social remittances constitute the
social practices, values, networks and resources that originate in the sending society
and are reconstructed in the receiving country. These are then transferred back to
the sending society, primarily via family visits 'home' and return migration. Social
remittances have the potential to transform society in terms of developing family
and community resources, business entrepreneurship and new ways of thinking
about society. But instead of pursuing these points any further here, we now turn
to a brief consideration of the boundaries and obligations of caring.

Caring boundaries and obligations

The reciprocal caring exchanges between transnational, inter-generational, and
intra-generational family members discussed here were based on personal networks established by families. Acts demonstrating caring for and caring about
were bounded by moral considerations and obligations that individuals felt that
they owed to family members. As we noted, expectations were gendered, with
women expected to subscribe to particular norms and values. For example, Anna
in Peterborough felt that she was morally bound to provide family care, and that
her identity as a woman would be affected if she failed to do so. Perhaps it was
this that led her to mistrust external agencies providing care:

Q: So it's 20 years that you began to look after your husband night and day?
A: Yes. If you don't wash his face he stays with a dirty face, if you don't feed him he goes without food, he doesn't ask for anything, you have to think things for him. I have to look after him always, night and day!
Q: And do you get any help from the council?
A: No! No! ... they always ask me if I want any help but thank God I always managed and I can still manage!
Q: You don't want help?
A: No!
Q: Why not?
A: Because I can manage, I don't need help.

(Anna, interview location: Peterborough, March 2004)

Anna's experiences illustrate Finch and Mason's (1993) notion of 'kinship morality' and the fact that a set of moral discourses informs our behaviour towards kin. As Williams suggested (2005), individuals are wont to negotiate their relationships within these moral guidelines and according to particular contexts.

In both studies young people's expectation of caring responsibility and the sense of obligation they felt towards their parents were openly discussed, and they all said that they would contribute towards care provision when their parents became older and/or experience ill health. Although their justifications varied as to the reasons why they would provide care, common themes running throughout the young people's accounts were to the effect that 'it was the right thing to do', they 'owed their parents', 'it is expected' of them, 'no other option', 'it's not even up for discussion', and 'it's a given, I will do it'. It could be suggested that the young people's strong sense of personal obligation and expectation to provide care for their parents was based on the expectation that children will reciprocate parents' sacrifices when bringing up their children. This behaviour is typical of what Komter (2005) described as 'delayed reciprocity'.

In contrast with young people's accounts, older respondents had direct experience with caring for sick and elderly parents and they described the tensions, burdens and feelings of guilt that their sense of moral obligations brought them. Perhaps because of the distance between aspirations of performing in the future according to a moral code, and the actual experience of struggling with the difficulties of delivery, we found that the expectation and obligation to care were much more muted among older respondents when compared with young people's accounts.

While there were many similarities between our Caribbean and Italian respondents, there were also some significant differences. For example, many Caribbeans did not consider it an unconditional or unquestioned duty that they be automatically responsible for the care of elderly parents or elderly relatives. These respondents took a much more pragmatic approach to their contributions to family care provisions. Their involvement in care provision reflected changing moral and cultural values as well as the contexts in which they found themselves. The strength of their particular kinship connections, the consideration of the needs of others in their family unit or household, and the social and economic resources that they had available at any given time were important considerations. These individuals were much more pragmatic and perhaps also more practical and realistic in assessing their capacity to reciprocate care.

In Italian families norms and obligations towards elderly care were less negotiated and less linked to past experiences of care than in Caribbean families. For example, both Marta and Silvia, professional women born in Britain, felt an obligation to care for their parents even though they felt neglected as children by their parents and had several problems with them when they were young. The notion of 'prescribed altruism' – that is the strongly felt inner norm of being obliged to demonstrate solidarity with aged family members (Finch 1993) – seems relevant for interpreting these Italian family practices.

In both studies, however, the main beneficiaries of care in later years were family members who had provided needed care to children or young adults. The care provided by younger people for the elderly were not always for their own natural parents. For example, Jocelyn was a retired grandmother who spent half the year in Britain and the other half in Guyana. As a child Jocelyn lived with her aunt and at the time of our interview she helped to care for her aunt by giving her money to pay for medical bills and dialysis treatment. Jocelyn also bought her aunt a blood pressure monitoring machine, and arranged for a live-in nurse to stay with her aunt. The interesting point here is this: Jocelyn's natural mother was also ill, but Jocelyn chose not to contribute towards her mother's care; this is because Jocelyn did not have a sense of obligation or responsibility to care for her mother. The fact that Jocelyn provided care for her aunt while doing nothing for her mother caused some tensions between Jocelyn and her family and a family rift occurred between her aunt and Jocelyn's mother, so that they were no longer on speaking terms. Similarly, another respondent, Latoya, recollected that her mother funded her brothers' visit to Britain so that he could receive hospital treatment because when Latoya's mother was a child her brother had cared for her and had also assisted her to migrate to Britain.

Thus, complex negotiations occur in families regarding kinship responsibilities, such as care provision. Finch and Mason (1993) distinguished between explicit and implicit processes of negotiation occurring in family relationships concerning decisions over who will undertake caring work. Explicit negotiations signify and involve open and clear discussions, often referred to as a 'family get together' or 'family conferences'. Implicit negotiations involve decisions and negotiations that occur without open discussion. Explicit negotiations occurred more often in Caribbean families, and implicit negotiations were found more often in Italian families, although both types of negotiations occurred in Caribbean and Italian families.

Explicit discussions between family members either happen face to face or on the telephone (with individual family members or teleconferencing) and do not usually include all family members but a selected few (Finch and Mason 1993). In the Caribbean study, interviewees were able clearly to identify family members, or the 'key players', who were usually involved in this negotiation process. They also used family discussions to keep abreast of family events and strengthen kinship bonds. The 'key players' were generally family members who are regarded as the most respected and/or senior family members. Important factors for choosing the key players involved the inter-relating factors of age and gender (oldest male sibling); socio-economic status (affluent family member with most money and resources); or professional/educational status (most educated). It was noted that other family members are also involved in these discussions – although not necessarily as 'key players' – including those members in close contact with each other and those who live with or in close contact with the family members requiring care. Also present in these negotiations were the family 'link person'. This represents the family member who acts as the family conduit, passing information and news between family members and connecting those living in different part of the world or country. These family discussions were rarely egalitarian, whereby family members present have equal say about decisions. More often than not other family members are informed of decisions after the 'key players' have decided on a course of action. In addition, it was also highlighted that those family members involved in decision-making processes may not be themselves directly involved in the practical day-to-day aspect of care provision.

Implicit negotiations could be 'tacit' or unspoken agreements between family members and this form of negotiation occurs for a number of reasons. Firstly, there is the 'obvious' and 'taken for granted' person to provide help where necessary or needed; therefore the negotiations remain unacknowledged (Finch and Mason 1993). The statement by married couple Paolo and Marcella described how they became the family's main carers because they had no children themselves but had experience of caring for elderly relatives:

P: In 1960 we moved here … primarily because Marcella and I were getting married and I was looking after my mother when my father died and so I could continue to look after my mother when we moved into this big house …. We have no children but we believe we were destined to look after all the old people of the family because we looked after her mother and father and we looked after my mother and my uncle and older relatives we looked after.
M: We'd never dreamed that it should be any different really.
(Paolo and Marcella, interview location: London, December 2003)

In other family situations, the choice of this 'taken for granted person' could also depend on the person's seniority within the family, or their geographical distance to the relative in need. It should be noted, too, that implicit negotiations may involve decisions about care that were sometimes taken unilaterally by individuals to avoid potential conflicts with other family members.

Conclusion

In this chapter we have focused on the problems involved in families providing care across national boundaries, across generations, and we have also considered issues about gender. These are aspects of a complex set of relationships that may be becoming more common, as families are able to provide for each other across boundaries of every kind. In the next chapter we turn to consider the significance of maintaining identities and sometimes inventing these as the needs of families and communities change.

7 Continuity and invention of identities within families and communities

Introduction

In this chapter we broaden the discussion to outline social networks for the continuity and invention of new identities for transnational family members. The cross-ethnic networks and bonds, combined with continued transnational and kin connections to the country of origin, informs our understanding of ethnic identity among new communities in Britain as illustrated by the Caribbean and Italian transnational experiences. Important aspects of these experiences include individual persons' narratives of such complex forces as migration and settlement, transnational networks, racism and social exclusion. We suggest that young people's ties that are being created are likely to be less rooted in their ancestral homeland or familial country of origin and more influenced by the cross-ethnic bonds and multi-ethnic networks resulting from their everyday relationships and their contact with people spanning diverse racial and ethnic categories. Alongside these bridging and cross-cultural interactions, networks and relationships, broader patterns of globalization and diaspora also create spaces for the invention of new identities for individuals, families and communities. More specifically, in this chapter we organize our arguments around issues of identities as expressed in rituals, the reconstruction and maintenance of these identities, and issues of exclusion.

Identities, rituals and ethnic associations

Families of Caribbean and Italian ancestry whom we interviewed in different parts of Britain illustrate the general point that the family is a crucial site for the articulation of ethnic and national identities. These families are linked into networks that reveal the multi-stranded social relations and processes that link together, and simultaneously connect, Caribbean and Italian migrants and their offspring to two or more nation-states. The subjectivities and identities that emerge for these individuals were embedded in networks of personal relationships which were unconstrained and not defined by geographical borders or distance from family members. Many respondents claimed allegiance to particular cultural groups who were unrelated to their place of residence or these individuals' citizenship. In order to maintain (and sometimes construct) their identities these individuals drew on the multi-stranded social relations of their parents' and wider families' country of origin. For these individuals, their transnational family networks were central to the constructions of fluid and multiple identities, which were simultaneously grounded in their connections to parents/grandparents homeland as well as their localized surroundings in Britain. These transnational relationships reinforced the importance of movements backward and forwards, or return migration in terms of the maintenance of family networks. Participation in transnational family rituals, cultural practices and activities was a key means of maintaining understandings of ethnic identity, and notions of home and belongingness.

For instance, we observed that Caribbean migrants and their offspring tended to forge a collective identity as part of a more widely constructed diasporic identity. When defining their ethnic identity they often emphasized their familial and cultural connection to the Caribbean region as a whole, rather than to a specific country in the region. They tended to construct a homogeneous discourse about what it means to be Caribbean, and the wide range of countries which form the Caribbean were sometimes overlooked. This was also true for their understandings of much of the structural divisions that exist in Caribbean communities in Britain, such as cultural, racial, class and gender differences. When forging collective ties and reinforcing ethnic bonds, offspring of Caribbean migrants drew strongly upon the combined factors of local space of residence of their parents and themselves, transnational kinship ties, and the experience (or perception) of racism and social exclusion. Makesha made this point very clearly in her reply to a question about identity:

> I know that I'm British because that's what it says on my passport but I don't feel accepted in England because I'm black and I know that black people are treated differently here. We're made to feel that we're tolerated but not completely accepted and we're not treated equally. I always tell my friends, who are black, 'you lot go on like you're equal', I said, 'but you're not'. I have to try and drum it into their heads. I know that I'm not really Jamaican in the sense that I wasn't born out there but I still choose to identify culturally with them because my parents are Jamaican and everything done in a Jamaican style at home and so it's what I feel more comfortable associating myself with them.
>
> (Makesha, interview location: London, October 2003)

Another interviewee, Keisha in Birmingham, echoed these sentiments, when she told us that

> I don't get to see my aunt and cousins there [Jamaica] that much. We mostly keep in contact by phone or email. But my cousins in Canada I see them often. I would say my family is important to me. They give me my cultural identity, my Caribbean identity.
> Q: How do you define a Caribbean identity?
> R: That's tricky one, I just am. It's who I am and my way of being and I think it's my family that give my 'Caribbean-ness'. I'm not sure that word exists but you

get what I'm trying to say, don't you? My family make me the person I am today and my identity comes through that family history and cultural heritage. We live in different parts of the world but to me that's not important because we all identify with each other because of our history. We have a natural affinity, a connection that doesn't have to be explained. Just knowing that they're out there supporting me helps me to understand who I am. When we do meet up you wouldn't think that it's been ages since we last got together because we just pick up where we left off.

(Keisha, interview location: Birmingham, February 2004)

The family and transnational bonds were equally relevant for British interviewees of Italian backgrounds. While outside factors such as community organizations and religious bodies play an important role in maintaining Italian identity (see, for example, Fortier 2000), the family and transnational kinship ties were of particular significance. As noted in an earlier chapter, Italian respondents not only maintained strong links with their kin left behind but for many of them the frame of reference remained oriented towards 'home' in Italy. Again, as earlier noted, after several years in Britain they continued to maintain strong links with their villages of origin, usually through regular phone calls, sending letters and above all visits when extended families are reconstituted, single male migrants look for brides and local feasts are celebrated.

This membership to wider transnational kinship networks by our Caribbean and Italian respondents enable them to be part of globally dispersed family networks, which cross generational and cultural divisions. These transnational kinship networks were generally considered to be supportive by our interviewees because, to varying degrees, they encouraged the maintenance and transmission of values, practices and identities within families and communities. Family networks were largely sustained by the participation of individual family members in family activities, rituals and ethnic-specific community associations. Within the family home, moreover, cultural signifiers were utilized by family members as an important social resource for the maintenance and transmission of cultural identities, values and practices.

Family rituals and celebrations also provided a key opportunity for transnational links to develop between family members residing in various parts of the world. It was evident in speaking with our respondents that family rituals played an important role in bringing distant family members together and reaffirming continuity of identities. The rituals that people participated in ranged from everyday activities, such as the manner in which the family meal was taken, to the cyclical festivities in the calendar year, such as Christmas and Easter celebrations. These also included life-cycle events, such as weddings, funerals and anniversaries. Jennifer, the offspring of Caribbean migrants, described the family reunions she attended and how individuals from different countries used these events to meet distant family members. Indeed, the principal aim of these reunions were to strengthen family ties and connections that were sometimes weakened or lost, despite family members' best efforts to maintain them (Sutton 2004). Jennifer told us that her mum's family held a family reunion in Texas in 2001 and I went with my mum and my sister. I was introduced to loads of these families that I didn't know existed. That was the first time I realized how big my mum's family was. Before that reunion I only knew about a few great aunts and cousins in Barbados but I had never met them before. Going to the reunion made me feel part of the bigger unit. Family came from all over, there were my cousins from Barbados and St Vincent, loads of family that live in the US and there was the European side of family. I met Leila there. She's a distant cousin who lives in Zurich. We hit it off straight away and we kept in contact with each other by emails. She comes over to visit a few times with her family and I've been over to Switzerland on a family visit. To think that this time three years ago I never knew she even existed and now we're so close each other.

(Jennifer, interview location: London, January 2004)

The cyclical events of Christmas and Easter provided our participants with the opportunity to celebrate Caribbean or Italian social and cultural practices, and in doing so reinforced their respective understandings of belongingness and collective membership to their ethnic groups. Many of the Caribbean respondents highlighted the importance of Christmas and Easter as festive religious periods when family and kinship members, who were globally dispersed, come together to reaffirm kinship ties. In celebrating such events together, these communities were able to take advantage of commonly shared practices with the majority societies. Andrew's testimony richly illustrates this point:

We have Christmas at our house, and it's my wife, her parents, my brothers and sisters and my parents and whichever uncle or aunt that happens to be visiting that year from America or the Caribbean. You've got all the phone calls, and you've got everybody ringing round to say 'Happy Christmas' to everybody in England and overseas. The phone calls are mainly to the Caribbean and definitely family in America. We buy those calling cards, you know the ones that cost £3, and we take it in turn to call around. The phone calls take up most of the day because some family we haven't spoken to for the whole year and we spend the time catching up on news and then passing it on to other family, so by the end of the day we all know what everyone else is up to. We also use email and last year we used Instant Messenger and we attached to the PC so we could speak to my cousins in Toronto in 'real time' and we could see them as we were talking. So that was something different, [it is] another way to get that closeness. And then Boxing Day, we'd have close family over to our house again because some family are Jehovah Witness and then that following weekend we would go over to our granddad's house, and it more family again. Then New Year's it's my cousin's house in Maidenhead, and another round of phone calls to say 'Happy New Year', so we do family things like that at Christmas.

(Andrew, interview location: London, January 2004)

Michael's account is equally revealing. Of Caribbean background, Michael highlighted how Christmas is utilized as an important social resource by the young people in maintaining inter- and intra-generational and cross-cultural family connections and relationships. He told us that his

> family is very close because we make the effort to stay in touch ... I always
> make sure I go home [to Jamaica] for Christmas. Usually about five or six of
> my 10 uncles and aunts go home. It's a family tradition that we meet up at
> my parents' house in Kingston and then travel down to my uncle in MoBay
> [Montego Bay] on Christmas Eve. Usually my uncle from Germany is there
> as well. Last Christmas, my aunt from New Zealand came. Some of my dad's
> aunties from the States were there, and three of his cousins and their kids, they
> all live in Canada. What we do when there is pretty much sit down and eat,
> drink and catch up with each other. Our family 'get togethers' are important.
> It keeps us emotionally close. I'm going to continue that with my children.
>   (Michael, interview location: London, March 2004)

In Michael's case, the relative ease and affordability of air travel meant that it was not too difficult for geographically dispersed family members to come together in the Caribbean. This reinforced Michael's ethnic and family ties to the region. The emotional bonds and connections that emerge through family and kin-based networks are not constrained by geographical or physical distance and national boundaries. In this sense the role of Christmas in maintaining these transnational emotional bonds mean that the festival became a signifying practice, invested with emotional meaning and defined by emotional ties and relationships of trust and reciprocity.

Other Caribbean offspring also discussed the customs and traditions that they followed on Christmas Day, but they were uncertain whether these customs and traditions were particular to their own family or represented wider aspects of their ethnic and/or national identity. Customs and family practices such as late Christmas brunch, an evening dinner, saying grace and blessing the table at mealtimes, visiting family and kinship members on Christmas night and Boxing Day, watching television programmes such as *EastEnders* and *Only Fools and Horses*, appeared to have become typical ritualized events commonly described in these respondents' accounts of Christmas. Our conversation in London with Marsha is an apt illustration of this point; she stressed that she

> usually help[s] mum do the breakfast or lunch, 'brunch' as she calls it! We have
> traditionally Guyanese food, pepperpot, garlic pork, salad and 'hard-dough'
> bread; well that's Jamaican but we've appropriated it as Guyanese! Lots of
> bucks fizz and sparkling wine. So we'll eat and whatever, and then we'll have to
> clear the table, stack the dishwasher, then the presents. After all the presents are
> opened, we clear up again. We'll lay the table for dinner. The kids'll be going on
> about when they can open their presents – this is every year – and they always
> ask, even though they know they can't open it until we've finished eating. Mum

goes in the kitchen, puts on her gospel music and starts cooking. And me and my dad help out wherever we're needed. And then my godmother comes with my cousins and she'll help to cook the dinner; it's a strictly unspoken thing, it just happens every year. My godmother comes with her presents for the kids, and they're like, 'Oh, more presents!' kind of thing! After the presents are opened we sit down to our main meal.

Q: What do you eat here?

A: Nothing special. The usual things like everyone else eat on Christmas Day. Macaroni and cheese, turkey, fish and lamb, rice and peas, and plain rice, vegetables, and plantain, gotta have plantain! And then we sit down to watch, whether it's *Only Fools and Horses*, or waiting to watch *EastEnders*, eating our dessert while *EastEnders* is on, and then after *EastEnders*, I watch a movie and then we're going out to visit my cousins.

(Marsha, interview location: London, April 2004)

Our Caribbean respondents identified a number of other Christmas customs and traditions practiced as ethnic-specific. For example, the practice of going to church on Christmas morning was considered by many young people to be typical of Caribbean cultural identity. Their understanding was framed by a cultural and historical context wherein Christmas is regarded as an important religious festival in the Caribbean and the practice of church-going and collective worship represents an important characteristic of Caribbean life. In Nottingham, Natalie told us that

On Christmas morning we all go to church; I'm not sure why but it's just family tradition. They used to do it back home [Caribbean] because it was expected and they've kept that going with us. I think there's more of a cultural element in there as well, because essentially, West Indians are a lot more religious and church-orientated than white people. Even if we're not practising it all the time, I think, when it comes down to it, we're a little bit more spiritual, or church-orientated than the average British family, and we take that kind of Christmas aspect well a lot more seriously.

(Natalie, interview location: Nottingham: November 2003)

Although Christmas has emerged in recent years as an important celebration for people of Italian origin in Britain, this has not always been the case. For example, Donatella remembered how Easter was originally more important for southern Italian migrants, like her parents, and church rituals and special meals were passed down from her parents' generation to her and her sister. She noticed that as the years went by, Easter lost its salience for her family and the status of Christmas changed and became the main celebration, largely for economic reasons. For many recently arrived Italian migrants to the UK, little money was spent on Christmas festivities primarily because all financial savings were directed to the August visit home.

For those families who became relatively better off, Christmas was a time of the year for conspicuous consumption and family togetherness. Special food and meals were prepared and gifts exchanged. Gender differences became part of the organization of Christmas events, with men involved with the shopping (under the women's guidance) and women concerned with the cooking and organization of specific events. Women in the family were, however, not equally involved in these events. There seemed to have been a 'natural' organizer, a person whose role was to make sure other relatives attended, making her house available to visitors, and doing the bulk of the cooking. Sometimes these tasks were shared among a small group of women, who undertook these tasks in turn or sometimes worked together. There seemed to be power attached to the organization of these events, usually in terms of prestige or influence. In some cases the rituals took place in the household that had the largest dining room (which often meant the wealthiest family in the kin group). Despite the changing nature of Christmas and Easter in Italian families, the one thing that remained consistent over time has been that these occasions were characterized by family reunions, the preparation of special food and meals. As in Caribbean communities, these occasions involved church attendances for British Italians, and therefore reinforced or maintained traditional values and norms.

In general, perhaps a more important way in which families and communities were brought together and reinforced their links with the 'homeland' and specific Italian identities were through life-cycle rituals such as baptisms, confirmations and weddings. Some of our respondents used such rituals as a way of bringing together scattered family members, whereas others use them as occasions to strengthen their links with their specific local 'Italian community'. This was the case in the close-knit Italian communities in places such as Bedford and Peterborough where weddings since the 1980s have become very large affairs. The explanation given for the large size of these events was that it was traditional for everybody in the community to be invited. Others chose, however, to celebrate these events in Italy rather than in Britain as a way of reaffirming continuity with their families' places of origin. This was the case for Francesca from London, who remembered that

> friends tended to have these … like First Communion or Confirmation in England with other Italians in an Italian church but in my case we went back to Sicily on both occasions and my mother was very insistent and wanted it to be in the church where she got married.
> Q: Why do you think that is the case?
> A: I think it's that continuity that is important to her in terms of where she was from and where she perceives … wanted us to locate ourselves in terms of where we belonged and up to that point, up to when I had my Confirmation, there was still this sense that we might go back. So I think it was partly to do with that and also I think her attachment is ultimately there and for me and my brother to continue that attachment was very important to her. I think that's why.
> (Francesca, interview location: London, December 2003)

Outside the sphere of family affairs, village patron day celebrations served to reaffirm ethnic identity in Britain. These celebrations remained important especially for the migrant generation, reminding them of their connections with their village of origin and of positive memories about their youth. Migrants were the main supporters of these village festivals, and they sent money to support these events and sometimes visited in order to participate. Interestingly, we noted that these celebrations had also changed and adjusted to accommodate the needs of migrants who were participating. For example, in Ribera organizers changed the procession time to fit in with a new TV connection with Riberesi associations in Canada and New York. We also noted that some of these 'village celebrations' were invented, adapted or imported. For example, in Carisolo the 4 July celebration became the main celebration in the village where emigrants to Britain and North America met and shared their experiences.

Participation in a number of community activities were therefore of significance in retaining ethnic identities. Two crucial examples were supplementary schooling and the black churches in Caribbean communities, and the participation of families of Italian backgrounds in churches and regional and other voluntary associations. Aspects of these have already been discussed in an earlier chapter, but we want here to emphasize the roles of supplementary schools in Caribbean communities and the churches in Italian communities.

Caribbean communities first established supplementary schools (held during the evenings or on a Saturday) during the late 1960s and the early 1970s. These schools were largely set up in response to parental dissatisfaction with the education system where a disproportionate number of black children were concentrated in what were termed educational sub-normal (ESN) schools (see, Goulbourne 2002, ch. 4; Goring 2004). The black supplementary school existed outside mainstream educational institutions and represented a form of self-help in Caribbean communities to counter the negative effects of mainstream schooling and raise the educational standards of their children (Callender 1997; Reay and Mirza 1997). Several decades later, the black supplementary school continues to represent an important aspect of Caribbean community life. In addition to academic learning – principally focused around reading, writing, arithmetic, black history and cultural studies – black supplementary schooling promoted Caribbean cultural traditions and values that further bind the young people to a Caribbean ethnic identity. Some Caribbean offspring attended black supplementary schools as children and some of them now teach in these schools. These respondents described ways that a shared Caribbean cultural and ethnic background encouraged mutual trust between teachers and parents. They also highlighted the sense of obligation and responsibility they have in being role models for Caribbean children, the desire to give back to the community and the importance of using a range of teaching styles and practices with which children of Caribbean origins could culturally connect. Karen spoke positively about her experience in this kind of community work when she told us that she

> wanted teaching experience. I wanted to work with black children to help educate them and make a difference. The Reverend Gregory, he said the spirits told him I'd make a good teacher. The parents would like me also because I

could relate to them. There were all different black teachers here, and I'm like, 'Oh, this is really nice, I belong here.' And it was so warming to see so many little black faces, you know. And being at the school is about putting back into the community because I'm doing something for my own people. So this is why I would always give up my Saturdays just to be here, and I don't even look at it as giving a Saturday, because I like being here.

(Karen, interview location: London, October 2003)

Like the black supplementary school, black-led churches are a long-established institution in the Caribbean community, representing a rich site of bonding social capital. During the early migration years, the period from the late 1940s through to the late 1960s, Caribbean migrants feeling increasingly excluded and marginalized in mainstream churches turned to the black-led churches that were emerging in major cities throughout Britain. Black-led churches also acted as a primary site of resistance for the Caribbean community against institutionally racist practices. Goulbourne (1989: 98) attributed this growth of black-led churches to three factors (i) the majority white society's rejection of black Christians and the different forms of worship in black congregations; (ii) class differences between practising white Christians (largely middle-class) and the majority of practising Caribbean migrants (largely working-class); and (iii) 'the evangelicism' of Caribbean Christians, irrespective of their denominational affiliation and conviction. These church congregations were overwhelmingly comprised of adult women, usually accompanied by their children. When these children reached adolescence their church attendance declined, but in the last decades they have witnessed, and in some cases experienced, a 'religious revival'. It is not surprising, therefore, that these churches have a strong youth membership. Talking to Caribbean offspring made it clear that black-led churches represented a key focal point for civic participation, structured youth activity within the Caribbean community, and the transmission of cultural values and practices, as the following conversation illustrates:

Q: Do you belong to any organizations or societies?
A: Black ones. Yeah. Mainly 'BYG' [black church youth group] is where most of my efforts go. The church is black-led. I also do a couple of things with the 'Seymour Fellowship' [training and mentoring programme].
Q: And why are you involved in these organizations?
A: I've grown up with black, white, or Indian or whatever. But it is important for me to see black role models. I do treasure the fact that I see people who look like me, doing the things that I might want to do. So that is definitely important. My dad has always been very into his black issues and black self-help. He feels it's important to support your own community. His ways have definitely rubbed off on me.

(Anthony, interview location, London, April 2004)

His father was an important spur for Anthony's active interest and participation in the black-led churches, but in general the social networks of Caribbean parents were instrumental in determining their children's identity and the type of activities in which they involved themselves. For example, parents who participated in other ethnic-specific organizations, such as the supplementary schools movement, were more likely to succeed in instilling in their children a sense of ethnic identity and utilize available resources in child-rearing contexts to do so.

Our Italians respondents were also deeply involved in a variety of associations, welfare organization and churches that offer services and information to UK-based people of Italian origin. These are usually divided into two main camps, reflecting divisions in Italy – Catholics and left-wing trade union groups. In spite of the apparent differences, both types of organization ran similar activities targeting the same groups of Italians who could participate in each set of events on different days of the week. In the sphere of elderly care, for instance, both Catholic and left-wing groups organized informal weekly meetings that functioned as day centres for retired Italians. Many of our interviewees were actively involved either as volunteers or simply as participants in these organizations, because of a sense of solidarity with other Italians who may have been in need; participants also felt that these gave them a sense of sociability and self-fulfilment.

One example of a social association for elderly Italian migrants is the drop-in centre in Peterborough funded by the county council. Italian groups had a booked slot once a week to which they were brought by mini-buses, and had a lunch. While there were about 100 members, on the days we attended there were usually around 50 members present. Generally, the men gathered in one corner playing cards while the women occupied the other side of the hall chatting or helping with the cooking. At lunchtime they all came together to partake of a simple Italian meal. When there were particular occasions to celebrate, some individuals brought something special, such as cakes or drinks, to share with their friends. Besides socializing and spending time with each other, the day at the centre also gave them the opportunity to ask questions and gather information about public matters that might affect them, such as pension and other entitlements.

Similar groups were active in Bedford and London, but in the capital there were also Italian women's clubs. Although these associations were opened to people from different age groups and social classes, attendance appeared to have been mainly by the elderly working-class people. This was true for several of the regional associations despite their efforts to recruit younger members. These centres and associations, as well as the church more generally, provided opportunities for socializing and passing time for the elderly. Those migrants interviewed in towns where these centres and associations do not exist (for example, Oxford and Aylesbury) felt more isolated. Many elderly Italian men in Oxford would meet in the mornings at the centre of a shopping mall, replicating the southern Italy experience where men would habitually meet in the central village square. As in southern Italy, women were excluded from such public spaces and gatherings and they were expected to stay at home; these events or moments were exclusively for the men.

One of the questions we asked interviewees was what it meant to be Caribbean and Italian and the ways in which they distinguished themselves from others. Some of what we have discussed so far revealed that both groups had relatively clear senses of what they thought distinguished them, but it is useful to explore a little further how they responded to this question in terms of their perceptions of themselves and how they conducted their lives.

Irrespective of age and generation, British Italians pointed to the importance of what they saw as the dense and close-knit family network, sitting down for meals as a family at least once a day, spending holidays and celebrations with family members as important distinguishing marks about themselves. They stressed the value of solidarity and cooperation among kin and to some extend among *paesani* (people from the same village) and co-ethnics. Although these aspects of identity were changing, they were underpinned by norms that were still strongly felt. When, for example, Francesca talked about helping family and community members she saw this as a trait of her Italian identity:

> It's a very positive thing that I'm able to not be completely selfish. I remember when my father went into hospital some people were saying 'Why do you have to go every time?' For me it would be bad not to go. This is very Italian that yourself is part of an extension of something very bigger like THE FAMILY.
>
> (Francesca, interview location: London, October 2003)

We have already seen how important the ritualization of food was to both cultures, but it appeared again and again as a signifier of identity. Of course, food has long been recognized as significant in health studies, economics, the sociology of religion and anthropology, and other fields, and so it was not surprising that food was perceived and consumed as an artefact imbued with social values and identities. Specific food items, the manner of their preparations, times of consumption and so forth reaffirmed aspects of cultural norms and ethnic belongingness across time and space. For example, many Caribbean respondents explained how important it is to 'season' or marinate fish a day or more before finally preparing it for eating. Many respondents talked about the importance of passing on knowledge to their children about the preparation and cooking of specific meals. Many of the women regarded this as an important part of their mothering practice and a way in which Caribbean culture is transmitted down the generations. Of course, some of these dishes such as the Jamaican 'rice and peas' (a misnomer) did in fact cross the Atlantic in different guises with migrants. But others (such as 'macaroni and cheese') have been the product of the imagination. In the Caribbean itself different countries and ethnic groups have their own distinct customary food dishes.

Of course, it is a truism that it is not possible to think or speak about Italian communities at home or abroad without food featuring as a central factor of identity. Rosanna's effervescence about her mother's nurturing practices through food and cooking is a strong testimony of this. Although they talked very little and had difficulties in communicating with each other, Rosanna was able to recognize and appreciate her mother's love and connection through her cooking. She told us that the only way she could really nurture us would be through her cooking and so I think in some ways I've kind of inherited that. I like giving pleasure through food to my family and I cook quite well because my mother is a fantastic cook, even by Italian standards. People always say 'Oh your mother, no one can cook like your mother' and one of the things that I regret is not writing it all down. What I'd like to do is maybe collect all her recipes through word of mouth because my brother has got them all up here [head]. He's a very good cook. I would like to document it and just keep all her recipes somewhere because my nephews and nieces in Canada they really love all this sort of food. They want to know how to make things when they come over from Canada and I have to show them how to do things. It's really sweet because they really want to keep that sort of thing going so I will do that one day. I will carefully record everything and keep it for them.

(Rosanna, interview location: London, March 2004)

The 'family meal' served as a powerful ritual to reaffirm ethnic identity, and as collective memory had high significance for all respondents of Italian ancestry. Food was seen by many to differentiate themselves from the English. Giovanna drew on her son's school essay to highlight the differences between an Italian and English meal, thus:

He was only six at the time and his essay it was really interesting because it said 'Eating is very important because it brings people together and I notice that when I eat with my grandparents in Italy I can't hear myself eating and my grandfather is always shouting and people are always shouting around me and one minute somebody is shouting and then somebody is laughing' and then he said 'but when I go to the English grandparents at Xmas time, it is very quiet and you can hear the snow falling and the knives and forks' and that was his creative writing piece. I thought that was really perceptive because it was just the sounds are very different and that's how he saw or heard it as a child. It's true isn't it?

(Giovanna, interview location: London, May 2004)

It is ironic that while these respondents claimed that they followed Italian traditions by having a cooked meal for the whole family once a day, some family visitors from Italy noted how Anglicized their relatives in Britain had become. Family members in England were having sandwiches for lunch at school or at work, and only having a main meal once a day in the evening. The norm in Italy was for two such meals in a day.

Identity construction and social exclusion

The integration of Caribbeans into British society has been complex. Their prominent public profiles in sports, in the music and entertainment world and in general pictorial representations are significant achievements and suggest a high degree of integration. On the other hand, however, the majority of Caribbean migrants and their offspring have encountered many social and economic obstacles, and are generally regarded to be less successful than their cousins who migrated and established families in the USA (see, for example, Foner 1979; Vickerman 1999; Waters 1999). Caribbean communities in Britain tend to be among the most socially and economically disadvantaged, as several national and local studies have shown over the past four decades or so (see, for example, Daniel 1968; Brown 1984; Modood *et al.* 1997; Owen 1994). Not surprisingly, therefore, many interviewees of Caribbean backgrounds reflected this structural position as well as their deep frustrations with their conditions which they thought hampered their ambitions for economic success and inter-generational upward social mobility.

Roystone's story is indicative of the way in which some Caribbean offspring's racialized and pathologized status impacted on their understanding of home and belonging, and made them also question their full integration into British society. Although interviewed in Jamaica, he told us

> [I] was born in England but I always felt unwelcome in my own country, so I can't call England home, if you mean home is as a place of warmth and comfort. I never felt that because prejudice and discrimination was always there. I didn't go out of my way to experience it. In London you grow up constantly looking over your shoulder, when you're out on the streets you go out with your guard up. I used to instinctively wonder what's going to come at me next. ... I was always getting stopped by the police. That policeman who stops you for some so-called driving offence, I'd be thinking 'now is he in a good mood today or has he had an argument that morning with the missus and if so he's about to take it out on my black arse?' ... It's a fact of life for us that many people in England can never understand. They don't understand the realities of being a black man and the feeling we're not liked or wanted. I never felt comfortable in my own skin there [England]. Now here [Jamaica] I'm comfortable in my own skin. I'm a very hard worker, I can hustle for a living and if you come to Jamaica with that attitude to work hard there's more options here to build your own business. I'm in a better position now to invest in a future for my family.
>
> (Roystone, interview location: Jamaica, July 2004)

We observed that this desire among the Caribbean offspring to reconstruct a Caribbean cultural identity and cultural ties to the Caribbean region was largely a consequence of their feelings of exclusion and marginalization in British society. A Caribbean cultural identity appeared to offer our respondents a sense of 'belonging' and 'connectedness'. Like Roystone, many felt that this identity provided their families and communities with an alternative mode of solidarity under which they could unite and collectively challenge the inequalities and feelings of marginalization encountered in British society.

Although people of Italian backgrounds share much the same racial identity as the majority indigenous population, and are generally successful, many also expressed frustrations arising from their experience of social exclusion and marginalization. Donatella in London told us that she could

> remember going to an opening [of an exhibition] once. There was a woman there that John [husband] works with and he introduced me, 'this is my partner, Donatella', and we started talking and she's really snotty and she said 'Oh, you speak very good English!' And I remember saying, 'yes and I can write it too!' and that was only like four years ago! That example reminds me 'oh my God, yes I am different too', at that stage that room was full of white, English, middle-class people, and that did really served to remind me.
>
> (Donatella, interview location: London, March 2004)

Later on in the interview Donatella explained that her Italian immigrant family status also contributed to her 'outsider' identity:

> I think I'm solid Italian, you can tell, no one ever thinks I'm English. I've got to be something, so having that label validates you. It gives me that interesting edge. It's lovely to have that different culture to engage with, to visit, beautiful country, beautiful food, it makes me a more interesting person I think so for me, and it's who I am, it's what's shaped me, it's what's made me, even though who knows what kind of interpretation of Italian I've got within me? Maybe this is just a result of my life pattern, my life experiences, whether they're Italian I don't know, but I am who I am, certain smells I like, things, the way I dress, where I like to shop, so parts of me that are very Italian and I can feel that.
>
> (Donatella, interview location: London, March 2004)

Italian migrants' offspring also reflected on the difference between themselves and the indigenous majority British population. Although some chose to rebel, the majority of these interviewees felt duty bound to conform to their parents' belief and cultural values about such things as marriage, family solidarity and togetherness. For some professional women such adherence can involve them in complex questions about the interrelation between ethnic and class identities. For example, one of our interviewees, Francesca, told us how her commitments to caring for and keeping links with her family were interpreted in middle-class English circles as lack of concern for her career and professional advancement. Another respondent, Giovanna, stressed that the children of Italian immigrants were experiencing personal identity crises. This crisis was framed around being both English and Italian but often feeling excluded in each context. Giovanna reflected that she was brought up as Italian and she took great personal pride in defining herself as such, cultivating Italian practices and values. She was therefore angry to discover that during her visits to Italy she was not seen as Italian by her family there nor by the public. She told us:

> I don't have British citizenship so I still have kept my Italian passport and Italian

citizenship and I can't become a British citizen unless I give that up and I'm not prepared to do that because I don't see why I should! If I call myself Italian it doesn't ring true and people always say 'Yeah, but you don't sound Italian' and when I'm in Italy I say 'I'm Inglese' [English] and yet I'm not English because my family is not English. I don't know

Q: But do you feel Italian?

A: I do identify much more with the Italian ways of living and doing things but this is my life. My mother tongue is English but I don't identify with England so … I don't know?

(Giovanna, interview location: London, May 2004)

While young people from both sets of communities 'look back' to their parents' homelands when articulating their identities, it must also be stressed that their understandings of ethnic identity were contextual and revealed the complex negotiations involved in highlighting or downplaying the different dimensions of their ethnicity. As Marley told us:

I'll go to Notting Hill carnival and I'll have the Guyanese rag but on St Patrick's Day I might wear a clover because I'm quarter Irish! When I go on holiday out of England I say, 'I'm from England'. But if it's like a one-one conversation with someone I've become friendly with then I'll say … 'I'm European and West Indian'. I've had to report to the police before and because … I can pass for 'white' I just let them assume that I'm white … I think they might treat me differently if they knew I was black. I also subconsciously alter the way I speak to people usually depending on what their ethnic origin is. … If I'm with a white guy who's a bit cockney I'll probably emphasise my cockney part of speech. But when I'm with my Jamaican guys I'll probably emphasize my West Indian part of speech like 'wha gwan?' [what's going on or, what's happening?]. It's just something I do automatically.

(Marley, interview location: London, October 2003)

In other words, young people of Caribbean and Italian – and by extension young people in other new communities in Britain – are carving out multiple identities for themselves. On the one hand, they appear to be utilizing social capital within their families and kinship networks to reaffirm and sometimes create a Caribbean or Italian ethnic identity. At the same time, they appeared to be developing processes and social networks that allow them to create identities across ethnic/racial and national boundaries. Cross-ethnic based contacts were formed around regional, neighbourhood and racial ties, as well as personal relationships, friendships and peer group membership. Marley's description of his friendship network is illustrative of the process:

I've mainly met my friends through school and my interests and my closest friends are all different races. My three closest friends are all different: West

Indian and from a single-parent background, white, English and very middle-class and Filipino. I'm involved in the local asylum groups and I'm into ecology and environmental issues and I've got to make friends doing this.

(Marley, interview location: London, October 2003)

In contrast, Giorgio, of an Italian background, highlights how he utilized his cross-ethnic childhood friendship network ties as a social resource in reinforcing his Italian identity

Growing up in Bedford, okay. We went to the local schools. We had quite a mixture but not a very big mixture of people. There were a few Italians because we used to live in the area; a few Asians but not many Asians; a few Blacks and the majority of them (the others) were obviously English. The thing is that as you were growing up through school, although you would mix with mostly all the people from different backgrounds. We all became fairly good friends … it didn't matter where you came from but we were always regarded as being Italian. The Asians were always regarded as being Indian or Pakistani and the Blacks were always regarded as being West Indians.

(Giorgio, interview location: Bedford, March 2004)

Some respondents rejected claims of transnational, national or regional identity and instead preferred to adopt a supranational one. Cristina, for example, reflected that, because she was not white and thus not English, she therefore called herself European.

Q: Okay. How do you define your ethnicity?
A: (laughs). I'm not white (laughs). I consider myself to be European.
Q: Right. Why?
A: Because I'm not white! I think I'm more European. I'm not British and I'm not Italian, I'm in no-man's land! I go back to Italy and, obviously, I speak Italian with an English accent … you can't win so I say I'm European now!

(Cristina, interview location: London, April 2004)

Giorgio made much the same point, when he stressed that

We were always regarded as being Italian so we were never really recognised as being English. I think as we grow older we believe that we are Italian. And it was drummed into us that, you know okay you're Italian. So we had this very strong pride of being Italian and that's probably carried on through the whole of my life really although I must admit when we used to go back to Italy for holidays the people of my age group there would regard me as being English … you're living in England and you're regarded as being Italian and you go to Italy and you're regarded as being English! So there was a little bit of you know? You start thinking to yourself you know. We grew up like that and I think to this day we are like that. If we're in England we still feel passionate and proud of being Italian. And at the same time when you're in Italy, even though we've only been there for short periods of time, you regard yourself as fairly English but not fully if you know what I mean?

(Giorgio, interview location: Bedford, March 2004)

This kind of variation was not unusual. In different contexts respondents had different senses about themselves – many felt 'Caribbean' or 'Italian' until they visited or went to live in these respective countries and then at that point realized how 'British' they either felt or were regarded. The interview with Roberto strongly brought out this point:

Q: Right, so when you were young and you were going to all these Italian things you didn't mind … you liked that?
A: I loved it. I loved Italian. I was Italian and we used to go to Italian football matches and I just loved everything Italian when I was younger.
Q: So you were proud of that?
A: Very proud.
Q: You didn't want to be English at the time?
A: Not at all. Now I'm English [with conviction!]. After living in Italy I'm definitely English. Their mentality is completely different.
Q: So you got along with the other second-generation Italians in London?
A: Yes. We had the same mentality. We were all born and brought up in England with Italian parents.

(Roberto, interview location: London, February 2004)

The sense of unease in different locations was very significant for Marta:

I don't know, this is home [in the UK], it's got to be home, but when I go skiing [in northern Italy], I'm going home, but I haven't got a house up there so it's difficult, no this is home, it's got to be hasn't it?
Q: You tell me!
A: I don't know, I feel at home up there, I feel at home, but my house, my job, and everything's here so home's here.

(Marta, interview location: March 2004)

There were some differences in the ways in which identity choices were articulated through gender and social class. For example, young working-class people from Caribbean backgrounds were likely closely to identify with a stylized form of black culture strongly influenced by popular *genres* from the worlds of African-American cities as well as parts of the Caribbean. For example, the type of music that was viewed as representing black youth cultural identity ranged from UK Grime (fusion of hip-hop, garage, RnB, reggae and house from the USA and Jamaica); Dancehall (fusion of reggae/roots from Jamaica); calypso (fusion of soca/steel drums from Trinidad and Barbados); UK Gospel (fusion of US Gospel and African oral narratives); and UK RnB (fusion of US Soul and hip-hop with UK northern soul).

The young people in the Caribbean study spoke of the pressure to conform to these hybridized images of black youth identity. They felt pressured to speaking in the 'right' way (that is, a stylized and adapted form of Jamaican Creole as well as slangs from the Caribbean); wearing the 'right' clothes (designer sportswear with Bling jewellery); and listening to the 'right' music (soul, rap, house, reggae). For girls, self-censorship in choice of dress was important, and again this was mostly influenced by rap and reggae music videos on MTV and other satellite channels. Much of this self-censorship was framed around dress codes and keeping within the confines and boundaries of what is acceptable and appropriate as the black youth dress code whilst not looking overtly sexual. Similarly, the young men felt under pressure to follow the mannerisms, gestures and fashion of rap/reggae artists (baggy, loose, sportswear appropriate names and brand trainers). There was also the pressure to have expensive accessories such as top-of-the-range mobile phones.

We tested the notion of shifting patterns of allegiance and cultural identification, and significance of generational differences with our respondents during the 2006 FIFA Football World Cup. Many English streets displayed the English flag of St George and the Dragon in support of the English national football team. The media welcomed the displays throughout England's towns and cities, because it suggested that the English national flag had been reclaimed from the political far right and was now truly representative of a new diverse multicultural England. We wanted to know whether new minority ethnic communities were participating in the celebrations of the flag and supporting the English team. After all, criticism was being levelled at the Scots and their relative failure to get behind the flag and support England in the tournament. Media debates similarly raised the issue of society's class divide concerning the prominence of the St George flag adorning people's houses in working-class neighbourhoods and its absence in middle-class neighbourhoods.

Travelling the streets of multicultural areas in London, we noticed that the St George flag was flying alongside an array of national flags from other parts of the world, suggesting that representation and loyalty in sports is a more complex matter for Britain's new minorities than Norman Tebbit pointed out some years ago. The English team was not always supported by members in the communities where we conducted interviews, but there were some supporters, influenced by considerations of dual and national identities, cultural and racial factors, the influence of family and friends, and admiration of the skills of individual players or other national teams.

Those of our respondents who fully supported England's success in the tournament identified that their support was based on the fact that England is becoming increasingly diverse, transforming itself from a monocultural to a multicultural society. The fact that significant numbers of black players are integrated into the national team also made it more acceptable to support England, as Winston told us: 'I support England. Gone are the old days when you never had any black players playing in the team, now there are lots of black players so it's now acceptable for black people to say they support England' (Winston, interview location: London, June 2006.)

The lack of support for England was based around notions of national identity and other cultural and racial factors. The Italian and Caribbean communities had different reasons for not supporting England. Italy, for example, has a longstanding and well-established football tradition, and enjoyed remarkable success at World Cup level. Therefore, among first-generation migrants and successive generations, support for the country of identification is very common, despite their being born in England or living here for many years. The case of Antonio, of Italian ancestry, was a clear example of this. Antonio spoke little Italian, lived in a leafy suburb of London, and all his friends were English. Yet, when it came to football, he did not identify with the English team and flag but was a strong supporter of Italy. He explained that with

> people like my friends for example, I say I'm Italian, I've had so many arguments with them cos like for football for example they say, you should support England, you're English, and I say I'm not, I'm Italian, there's no English blood in me, my blood is Italian, I happened to be born in England, but that don't mean I'm English, I may be British, but I can't say I'm English, they can't see it, they think if you're born in a country then that's what you are.
>
> (Antonio, interview location: London, June 2006)

As with many other Italian respondents, Marco was proud of his Italian roots and for him football was one of the symbols of what was good about Italy, as he told us:

> The football team, films, passion, food – all the good things come from Italy pretty much, like you look at all the great actors like De Niro, Brando, they're all Italian, all the best food is Italian, the fashion, Armani, Dolce & Gabbana, the best footballers, it's got to be Italy really.
>
> (Marco, interview location: Bedford, June 2006)

Of course, where football is concerned, the Caribbean is not in the same league as Italy. But the participation of the Jamaica team as the 'Reggae boys' in World Cup 1998 and the Trinidad team as the 'Soca Warriors' in a later World Cup meant that Caribbean nations were being noticed. Despite being 'underdogs' in the football world (or perhaps because of this), Caribbeans in Britain exhibited a strong identification with, and support for, any Caribbean country competing at world level. Their continuing experiences of racism and racial connections to the black dispaora also created for some of them a sense of moral obligation in supporting Caribbean teams, and also other black, African and Latin American (particularly, Brazil) football nations, over and above England. Marcus, even in a city such as Manchester, was firm in this view, when he told us that

> Anybody but England to win it, I don't care just as long as it's not England because they're too racist. There's a lot of politics that goes into making sure they've not got too many black players in the national side. It is unlikely that

we will ever see the English national squad completely made up of black footballers. The FA wouldn't allow that to happen with the national team. But I believe that a team like France, they pick their best players and if it means they play an all black football team then so be it. That's why France won the World Cup and European Cup in recent times because they choose the best players.

(Marcus, interview location: Manchester, June 2006)

Peter in London was even more forceful on this point; he stressed that 'I don't have anything against England, but I feel it is my duty as a black man to support all of the black teams from Africa and the Caribbean' (Peter, interview location: London, June 2006). Many British-born respondents and their children stressed that their friends and everyone around them were involved with football. On a general level, this suggests that family, friends, and cultural traditions are important in influencing people's choice in supporting sport teams. In some instances, failure to follow these traditions results in much censoring and criticism in families. A case in point was Marcella, an Italian living in England, who switched her support from Italy to England and thereby caused great consternation in her family. Discussing the views of her best friend and family about this shift of loyalty, Marcella told us that her friend

says I'm terrible and I'm not patriotic at all … She supports Italy in the football, she thinks it's disgusting that I support England and my brother thinks it's disgusting. My children too, they think they are Italian.

(Marcella, interview location: London, June 2006)

The Italian respondents sometimes also shifted their support between two countries or would support both Italy and England. Similarly for the Caribbean offspring, it was common for them to support both England and Brazil or shift between these two national teams, as Melinda told us:

I always support Jamaica. And then I always support Brazil as well. If England are playing another European side then I'll support England but not if they [England] are playing France and Holland because I support those team too.

(Melinda, interview location: London, June 2006)

Perhaps this difficulty in picking one team and fully supporting them throughout the whole tournament revealed the wider complexity of integration and what it meant to be truly multicultural, with shifting identities. The World Cup tournament provided an arena where some individuals rejected the idea of exclusively choosing one national identity over another. Instead, they simultaneously chose multiple identities, as reflected in their support of multiple teams, which was continually shifting and transgressing national boundaries.

Conclusion

In conclusion it is important to recognize that the changing contexts in which communities of Caribbean and Italian backgrounds in Britain define their ethnic identities reinforced the basic paradox of ethnic identity formation. Sometimes groups and individuals are wont to present and articulate ethnic identities as fixed, immutable and impenetrable boundaries. However, people's everyday lives tell a different story. Our respondents' accounts illustrated that ethnic identities are often fluid and mutable, and the construction of ethnic identities involve a continual negotiation around transnational family networks, communities, regional and diaspora racial connections.

8   Problems of belonging and 'return'

Introduction

Important and dynamic aspects of the lives of transnational families are the dreams and experience of return to an actual or a presumed homeland. While there may have long been dreams of return entertained by migrants, the forces of globalization discussed earlier make it increasingly possible for whole families or members to make the return a reality. Although from time to time in this discussion we have mentioned this phenomenon, in this chapter we examine more closely how the dreams and experience of return are articulated by transnational families.

Reasons for returning: the migrants

The literature on return migration explores the reasons given by a variety of migrant groups for returning (see, for example, King 1979, 2000; Gmelch 1980; Abenaty 2000; Carling 2002; Goulbourne 2002; Nathan 2007; Ni Laoire 2007). For example, in his review article on return migration, Gmelch (1980) identified four main reasons for returning. These include unfavourable economic conditions in the host society; strong family ties and migrants' desire to be close families and friends; feelings of loyalty to the home society; and push factors in the country of settlement, such as discrimination and racism. More recent studies have confirmed the importance of family ties in influencing return as well as in facilitating it (Reynolds 2008). In her study of returning Irish migrants Ni Laoire (2007) discussed, first, the role of obligation and family commitment (see also, Baldassar 2001; Carling 2002), and second, migrants' desire to return to a locality where they have access to a 'social field'. She defined this 'field' as the network of human resources that the migrants expect to be able to draw upon as well as contribute to, what in Part I of this book we described as social capital. Linked to this Ni Laoire (2007) identifies the desire to return to a safe haven, a place where migrants can cease to feel that they are outsiders (see also Reynolds 2008). Nathan (2007) in his study of health workers in Britain returning to Mauritius found that many migrants wanted to be assured within the settings of what they knew earlier in life as well as hoping for a better retirement in their homelands. In addition to these factors, Goulbourne (2002), pointed to a relatively new development in the Caribbean in the 1990s – the role of such pull factors in stimulating return, such as the help provided by governments to facilitate and make smooth the paths of citizens returning from abroad.

Others have explored the reasons why migrants postpone or fail to return. These include not having enough savings, not having a job and/or a home in the country of return, and finally, but perhaps most importantly, having emotional or social ties with the host society, especially through the migrants' children (Carling 2002; Goulbourne 2002). In her study of Italians in Britain, Ganga (2006) stressed that those who did not wish to return were concerned about care in their old age, and felt that this would be better provided in Britain than in their country of origin.

In order to understand how return is interpreted and lived by the people we interviewed, it is important to explain the contexts in which these have taken place. This means considering the migrants' original migration project and their views about what they thought constituted a successful migration experience. Caribbean migrants in Britain have always dreamt of returning, and this represented an integral feature of their migration experience. In many ways this is not dissimilar to the family narratives of other migrants, such as those from the Indian sub-continent, as Anwar (1979) argued with respect to Pakistanis. King (1979) noted that typical of the return migration process is the 'return' to the familial ancestral homeland. The collective migrant narrative shared by many in Caribbean communities in Britain is that many intended to stay in the receiving country for only a relatively short period of time in order to save enough money to return and financially establish themselves in their country of origin (Peach 1968; James and Harris 1993; Phillips and Philips 1998). However, for various reasons, including economic hardship, structural disadvantage and cross-generational family roots becoming firmly established in the UK, the plan to return was not realized for the majority of migrants.

Social resources and transnational activities were utilized by migrants to keep this dream alive in their own and their children's imaginations. Examples included the practice of writing letters and sending 'barrels' of goods to family members in the sending country; the prominent place of cultural signifiers and artefacts in the household to remember 'home' such as maps, sculptures, paintings, and items of furnishing; and the recital of Caribbean folk-stories and poems passed on to their children. These were forms of 'investments' for the future. But perhaps the most significant was investments in land ownership and the building or purchasing of houses for a future return.

In the remainder of this section, we draw mainly on our Italian data to illustrate the return of the migrant, because in general, Italian migrants seemed to regard return as an obligation. Baldassar (2001), in her study of Italian migrants in Australia, identified the 'obligation to return' as a key cultural value that underlies this group experience of migration. She saw migrants as having a 'licence to leave' their families in order to escape poverty, but also an 'obligation to return' when they had earned enough to be able to settle back in Italy. Baldassar also noted how migrants who settled permanently abroad had to justify their failure to return to their families and townspeople back at home. For Wessendorf (2007) 'the desire to return' was an important element in the construction of an Italian diasporic identity. Thus, Carmelo Petrucci, who returned to Ribera (Sicily) with his ice cream van in the 1980s, summarized how return was taken for granted when he said 'we are like elephants, we go back to die where we were born'.

Return has always been constructed by Italian migrants as the ideal scenario (King 1979; Wessendorf 2007). Baldassar identified Italian migrants, especially those who moved in the 1950s and 1960s, as homeland-focused (Baldassar 2007). Their migration plan entailed coming back to the village of origin with enough capital to buy a house and ideally become self-employed (King 1979). This orientation to the homeland led to many remaining ambivalent about belonging to the country of settlement and being torn between their responsibilities towards their children and grandchildren and their kin left in Italy.

An example from Sicily may be useful here. Many Riberesi returned in the 1980s at the time when the local economic situation seemed promising, mainly due to the production and commercialization of oranges. This cohort of migrants returned before retirement age after having lived between 10 and 30 years in Britain. They sold their properties in Britain and with the proceeds bought homes and land in Ribera, managing in some cases to set up a business in town (examples included a glass workshop, a shop, an ice cream van). The main reason for returning at that particular time was their attempt to fulfil their migration project, which meant returning to the village and resettling the *whole* family, owning their own homes, a piece of land and/or a business. Apart from the sudden economic boom in orange cultivation, the sudden return was also due to the fact that their children (especially daughters) had reached puberty. These migrants' main worry was that if their children were to marry in Britain (especially if they married outside Italian communities), their migration project of returning to the village as a family unit would become unattainable. As Giulio Martini, who was interviewed in Sicily in June 2005, explained, 'all the migrants had the plan to return and keep the family together'. He went to the UK in 1966 but said that he had always wanted to go back to his land. He and his brother decided to return when their children started elementary school. They feared that if they left it any longer they would not have been able to return as a family; he appeared to fear that 'the girls could have met English boyfriends and married in the UK'.

Unfortunately, things did not always work out as migrants from Riberesi had planned. Although most of them managed to return and buy properties, and in some cases set up businesses, their main goal of living in close proximity to their immediate kin proved difficult to achieve. It appeared that, in spite of all their efforts, transnationalism and migration, once set in motion are difficult to stop, and the economic boom in Ribera was short-lived. Competition from Spain and Morocco meant lowering prices for local oranges as well as difficulties in placing them in the northern Italian market. There were few alternative economic opportunities available in the town.

Consequently, after living a few years in Sicily, Guilio's daughters moved to northern Italy for work, which for him was 'the same as if they were abroad. This is the big *rammarico* [regret] we all have, having failed to keep the family united', as he bitterly remarked. Interestingly, Guilio did not see the social mobility that his daughters could achieve as a positive outcome of his own *sacrifice*;[1] he saw their departure as a failure of his migration project and of not having being able to set up the girls comfortably in their native Ribera.

Another interviewee, Maria, felt that she had also failed in her family project. She had returned to Ribera because her 18-year-old daughter 'didn't want to get engaged with anyone'. This meant that she did not want to marry someone from the local Italian communities in Britain. She did eventually marry a Riberese upon return but he was himself a returnee from Germany and they decided to settle their new family in Germany. Meanwhile, Maria's other daughter, who had married an Italian in London, continued to live there. Maria herself stayed in Ribera with her husband and her grandson, but when he turned 10 he too left her to reunite with his parents in Germany.

Even those who returned much earlier, mainly because they were unable to endure the hardship of family separation (Parreñas 2001), found themselves involved in long-distance or transnational family relations. In our interview with Anna in Sicily in June 2005 Anna explained that she had spent only five years in London, deciding to return even though she and her husband had not achieved any of their economic goals. She said that she convinced her husband to return because she could not continue to live apart from her two children whom she had left behind. She reported an episode when her son said to his father that he was not his dad, calling his grandfather 'Dad' instead. This episode, she explained, made her decide that it was time to return, but the family remained split, with Anna's daughter choosing to live in northern Italy. These developments caused Anna and her husband to think that if they had stayed in Britain they and their children would have remained together.

Among the Italian study participants only a minority returned upon retirement. Those who waited longer to return found it difficult eventually to take that step since such factors as family commitments, health considerations and so on had tied them to their country of settlement (Ganga 2006). Gabriella's parents were among the few able to fulfil the project of return upon retirement, partly because one of their daughters was already living in Italy. Their other daughter Donatella explained that

> My dad always said he had a life plan, he wanted to go home that's what he said and I never thought they would do it really 'cos they loved where they were. They felt quite comfortable but then my dad always had this thing, he wanted to go home.
>
> (Donatella, interview location: London, March 2003)

Return for Italian migrants mean returning to the village of their origins, close to the kin and friends from whom they had separated. This contrasts with Caribbeans, for whom successful return does not always mean going back to their local places of origins but, significantly, frequently resettling in different parts of their 'home' (Goulbourne 2002; Reynolds 2008). Returning Caribbeans often resettle in localities where they previously aspired to live but could not afford to do so before emigrating. For them upward social mobility, as reflected in residence, is an important part of their migration narrative and experience. This is also reflected in the huge houses they purchase or build, their cultivation of English lifestyles, such as afternoon tea, and other symbolic gestures that mark them out as having returned from England. Upward social mobility, however, is not the only reason for choosing to live in sought-after neighbourhoods. Some Caribbean families have to do so because family links have been lost in their places of origin (through mortality and migration to North America) or family obligations to those who are less well-off may be too demanding, or there may be the desire to live close to others who share aspects of a life in England.

For returning Italian migrants this would be seen as 'false return' and ultimately as a failure of their migration projects. The obligation to a specific locality was strongly expressed by Giovanni from Trentino:

> They offered me possibilities to start businesses in Genoa and Bologna but I said no, I'm not coming back to Italy if it's not somewhere near here. That was also my father's dream, that I would also came back near to home.
> (Giovanni, interview location: Trentino, September 2005)

Giacomo, also a Trentini, reinforced this point when speaking about working opportunities in other parts of Italy: 'If it would have been to go back to a city like Milan or Turin and start working there I would have said no, I would have never have gone to one of those cities' (Giacomo, interview location: Trentino, September 2005).

Giordana, whom we interviewed in Sicily in the summer of 2005, explained that she and her husband did initially return to Milan, where they both found work, but 18 years later (and before reaching retirement age) her husband 'felt the village call', as she put it, and they both went back to Sicily. This focus on the village of origins is crucial to their project of return. In the south of the country – as with the Caribbeans – they tended to build large houses to symbolize their upward social mobility; in the north, such public display of wealth was less common and returnees tried to fit back in the village life as if they had never left. Returnees in both south and north stressed their desire to go back to a community where they and their families were known, where family life could be enjoyed, the pace of life was slower, where social relationships were perceived to be stronger and where they felt they could cease to feel like outsiders to the society. Some returnees also stressed the importance of nature and the outdoor life – which were linked to their memories of childhood and youth, and sharply contrasted to the constraints of city life during their sojourn abroad.

Reasons for returning: migrants' children and grandchildren

As was to be expected, both sets of communities in Britain among whom we conducted interviews, revealed generational differences in their respective understandings of 'home' and 'belonging'. Naturally, and as we have seen, the migrants' understanding was influenced by memories of the country of origin and the specific place they had left behind. The experience of disruption and displacement caused by migration and of feeling 'alien' were at the forefront of their accounts. Their offsprings' understandings were shaped by their political positions on the questions of 'home' and 'belonging', and these were, in turn, informed by issues about exclusion, racism, their subjective positioning as the 'other' and their relationship with 'imagined communities' that represented a place often beyond their direct experiences. Some individuals of Caribbean ancestry identified themselves as belonging to a 'Caribbean' cultural landscape and viewed this as their 'home'. They valued the opportunity, where possible, to make family links and to visit the Caribbean for short periods, but did not express a desire to 'return home' on a permanent basis. These individuals regarded themselves as being at 'home' in Britain, while at the same time some of them also expressed the view that they did not feel they 'belonged'. For others, however, there was a strong desire to 'return' to the countries from which their parents came.

In recent years there has been a growing interest in offspring migrating to their parents' country of origin (Panagakos 2004; Potter 2005; Christou 2006; Wessendorf 2007; Reynolds 2008). But, as Goulbourne (2002) and Abenaty (2000) had earlier pointed out, strictly speaking this migration cannot be defined as 'return' because these offspring may not have lived in the country of their parents' birth. Moreover, as they both variously pointed out, some of the 'returnees' may not have had any ancestral connections with the country of 'return', because Caribbeans often have spouses from the majority indigenous European communities as well as other communities whose families may not necessarily be associated with the Caribbean. Some offspring and spouses were, however, familiar with aspects of the place of 'return', through taking holidays or, as we saw earlier, they had been sent to spend time with other family members. In addition, some young people would have partaken of their parents' conversations about their memories, nostalgia and longings about 'back home'. These narratives acted as important resources in building emotional attachments to the family homeland or country of origin, and sometimes influenced the decision to 'return' (see, Western 1992; Goulbourne 2002; Reynolds 2008). This kind of 'return' migration also reflects the transnational networks into which migrants' offspring are embedded and the personal and social relationships that connect place of birth, ancestral homeland and diaspora (see, for example, Levitt 2001; Foner 2002; Glick-Schiller 2004; Christou 2006; King and Christou 2008). The frequently repeated narrative of the hope that one day the family would return 'home' became part of offspring's earliest memories of family life. Wessendorf (2007: 191) defines this type of migration to the parental or ancestral homeland as 'root migration', highlighting this kind of migrant's 'search of a place which provides them with a strong sense of identification and belonging'. In this part of our discussion, we again draw upon our data from our Italian sample in order to illustrate the long history of migration and return migration that is common to both Italy and the Caribbean.

Most of the villagers of the Rendena valley, where part of our fieldwork was conducted are children of migrants or have had migrants in their families for the better part of a century. Mr Pollini, a returnee to the valley, claimed that as many as about 80–90 per cent of the population shared such a background. The original migrants left these impoverished mountain valleys at the end of the nineteenth century to work as itinerant knife grinders. Some managed to emigrate to the USA while others reached London on foot and settled there. Initially, only the men emigrated, leaving the women to look after the fields, animals and the numerous children born during the periodic visits of the emigrants. Subsequently, these men took with them their eldest children to help them in the businesses started; later, the wives joined their husbands, but men continued to return to the village for long periods at regular intervals. Siblings therefore started to be born in different countries, some in the village and some abroad, depending on where the family was at that particular time.

By the 1960s, some of the original migrants' offspring from Britain were marrying villagers while on holiday, and they returned to London. In addition, a new cohort of men left the still poverty-stricken valley in the 1950s, 1960s and to a lesser extent in the early 1970s. In addition to village women, sometimes these men married English women and sometimes the daughters of the original migrants for whom they often worked. For over a hundred years, knife-grinders emigrated from the Rendena valley, returned on holidays, or long visits, and in some cases permanently returned. In these circumstances, it's is difficult to speak about the different generations of migrants and returnees, because different members of the same family had different nationalities and experiences and where people happened to be born seemed in some cases to be fortuitous.

For example, Tom Pollini (interviewed in Trentino in September 2005) was born in Britain in 1922 of Italian parents, but, as he said, 'we grow up both in the UK and in Trentino, we spent long periods here, I have done elementary school here. This was common'. He added, 'there were many families coming and going'. He finished his studies and worked with his father in Britain, eventually 'returning' to Trentino in 1956 to open a bar with his wife (whom he had married during a holiday and who lived in London for just 18 months). His mother had already returned in 1947 but kept visiting Britain because two of her children were buried there (they had died during their internment as enemies of war on the Isle of Man). Asked why he had 'returned', Tom replied that 'we had a house here, sentimental reasons, memories, also of the grandparents, we grew up both here and there and we have always been in love with our mountains'. Tom's brother also returned in the 1970s. For his daughter Maddalena, who returned as a 13-year-old girl, the reason was that

> [in] 1970–1 they started talking about coming here and return[ing] to Italy because of the family, because there were still brothers and a sister here. I also think that mum and dad were a bit tired of the city. He loved his mountains, nature; he wouldn't move from this place.
>
> (Maddalena, interview location, Trentino 2005)

For her this planned trip did not feel like a return 'home' since she had felt fully English at school and well integrated there. Nonetheless, she was happy about the plan, having frequently been on holiday in the valley; as she recalled '[it] was very exciting, the house, nature, the walks in the mountains, things that there [in London] you were never doing' (Maddalena, interview location: Trentino, 2005).

Another example where migrant and returnee generations were difficult to differentiate was that of Giovanni Maturi's family. His grandfather migrated to the USA at the beginning of the twentieth century, and in the 1930s decided that his eldest son should join him to help with the business; but first he wanted his son to be fluent in English, to prevent his experiencing the problems of exclusion he himself had gone through; and so he sent his son to London, where Giovanni had a sister. When he returned to Trentino to prepare his son's trip to the USA Giovanni fell ill and died prematurely. His son stayed on in London and started working as a knife-grinder. Giovanni's father left for London in 1956 to go to work with his brother, leaving his family behind. Giovanni was then eight years old and his three sisters were respectively nine, three and few months old. In 1961 the family was reunited in London. Giovanni went to school there until he was forced to leave his successful studies to go to work with his father, who had become ill. During the 1970s he helped his parents build a house in Trentino. His father, however, died on their first trip to the new house and Giovanni, his wife (whom he had met during a holiday in Italy), and his mother decided to stay in Trentino for the sake of family. Giovanni explained that his mother 'wanted to stay in the new house in Italy but she felt the obligation to keep on coming to London because I was there. I felt I was slowing down everybody, so I decided so be it, I will return' (Maddalena, interview location: Trentino, September 2005).

Although Giovanni was not born in Britain, he was called 'the English' by other Italian youths because of what was regarded as his 'good' English accent and the manner of his integration in the local community as a youth councillor.

Carmelo's family narrative is equally interesting and complex. His grandfather went on foot to London in 1901, and his son (Carmelo's father) joined him in 1913 at the age of thirteen. Carmelo's father married a woman from his family's village in 1930, and she joined him in London, where Carmelo was later born. In 1966, Carmelo himself married a woman from the same village, who naturally joined her husband in London. As a child Carmelo visited Italy regularly, and he remembered the whole family's first visit in 1947 for six months. In subsequent years one family member or a business associate would visit on a three-yearly cycle so that the business would not be disrupted. Carmelo explained that 'one year would go my father, then my brother, then it would be my turn'.

In some cases, as in the Petrucci family, it was the wife from Italy who pushed for the return home. These wives found it difficult in the first years in Britain, socially isolated with young children and spending a lot of time alone in the house. For example, Mrs Petrucci retained positive memories of her village, which offered a better quality of life (even if economic prospects at the time were lower), and therefore a better place to bring up their children. This narrative resonates with Ni Laoire's (2007) observation that the desire for return is often coloured by memories of an idyllic rural childhood, even when the decision to return may have been motivated by such broader factors as family lifestyles, the need to draw upon family social capital, or to fulfil family obligations.

For younger people who returned in the last decade or so, Italy at times represented a safe haven in times of crises, or a place where to run to away from family problems in the diaspora. This was so for Joseph Sartorelli. He fell out with his brother, with whom he shared the family knife-grinding business in London. His father had already returned to his native village and Joseph decided to stay on there after a visit. At the time of interview, he worked seasonally in tourism and was still thinking about what to do next. Some women claimed that they ended up in Italy almost by chance, but actually their return was motivated or facilitated by their strong transnational practices and connections. Marcella, for example, told us that her return

> happened by chance. I had a friend ... we went to school together and she emigrated to Italy. Now my mum comes from Trentino and my father comes from Emilia and she emigrated to Piacenza and I used to work for British Airways so it was very cheap to go and travel and we were quite good friends. So, I went over and we formed a gang ... you know what it's like in Italy? ... You have your *compagnia* [groups of friends] and it was lovely and we went to a nightclub and my [future] husband used to be in nightclubs and I met him and after six months we got married.
>
> (Giovanni, interview location: Trentino, September 2005)

Others deliberately chose to marry in Italy as a way of getting away from the close-knit family and community in Britain while at the same time not disappointing their parents. The experiences of these wives were usually rather negative, as we will see later, and for Marta the escape turned on itself, as she explained:

> I really wanted to go and live in Italy, I wanted to get away from ... not my mum, but you know, mothers are very ... The boys are fine, the boys can do anything and everything, the girls can't do nothing! So I thought, yeah get married, go and live in Italy, but it didn't work like that, he got made redundant, or he got the sack and he came and worked over here for a year before we got married and lived in our house.
>
> (Marta, interview location: London, 2004)

Although we have not drawn here on our Caribbean data, there were similarities between the Caribbean diaspora and the Italians. As Potter noted: 'return migrants are best viewed as people endowed with social capital, potential and realized' (Potter 2005: 14). Certainly, the analysis of the Caribbean data indicates that for those who have taken the decision to return to the Caribbean, this migration is facilitated through the social relationships and resources that are generated and sustained through their family networks. It is these family networks which make the difference between the dream or intention to return and the actual reality of doing so. The Italian illustrations as well as other studies also highlight that strong family ties and strong connections to the family homeland provide the primary reason for return over and above other economic, social and political considerations (Gmelch 1980; Foner 2000). The main difference between the two groups has to do with the prospects of social and above all economic benefits of return, as we describe below.

Experiencing the return: the migrants

Although in general migrants wished to return, for many the actual experience of return was less straightforward than they had anticipated. Not surprisingly, there were variations in the return experience according to gender, the time of return, the economic situation in the place of return, and so forth. In this part of the discussion we again draw on the Italian example to illustrate how some returnees expressed their experiences on the return to the starting points of their sojourn.

As one would expect, the men seemed to adjust better to the return. In Sicily, they kept busy by joining other elderly men in the central streets cafés and working the land as a pastime. In Trentino they had meetings in bars and went for walks in the mountains. In contrast, the women suffered from the loss of gender autonomy, particularly so in the case of Riberesi women who had worked when they were abroad. Many encountered 'culture shock' moving from the city back to the village, with its strong social control. The women missed their homes in Britain, and generally complained about life in small Italian towns. They resented the gossip, felt they had fewer places to go to or things to do, and had no weekly meetings at social centres as they had in Britain. The anonymity of large department stores, where they could go shopping or simply pass their time with their friends, were missing. At the same time, both men and women longed for past times in Italy during their youth when – at least in their memories – people spent more time together, helped each other and TVs and modern life had not pushed everyone to lead isolated lives. At the same time they lamented the lack of privacy that came with the village life, hated the pressure to conform to norms they no longer shared, and struggled to adjust to the chaotic Italian bureaucratic system and ways of doing things. Giuseppe told us that

> what they found hard was the system, so the system wasn't ... and my dad became very Anglicized, he would queue for hours, he knows how to queue, he likes to queue, he likes to wait, in Italy they don't do that, just simple things you know, he likes form filling my dad, there aren't forms to fill you just pay a bribe, so he found all the bureaucratic system very difficult to adjust to.
> (Giuseppe, interview location: Sicily, June 2005)

Giuseppe said that both men and women felt like 'fishes out of water', and they therefore tried to preserve objects and habits that symbolized their previous lives in Britain. For instance, Francesca proudly showed her floral carpet from the 1970s with which she covered her flat in Trentino, explained that this was the original carpet she had in her London home which she greatly missed. Maria had two large tea pots very visibly placed on the stove in her kitchen in Sicily. When we visited her she offered tea, claiming that was what she always drank, and that it was brought back directly from the UK. She liked to get 'English' food that she missed, such as baked beans and bacon, from UK visitors. In spite of having complained for years about the inferior quality of English food, once back in Italy, many returnees longed for it, so much so that local shops in Ribera started to sell a variety of items popular with returnees. Another interviewee, Tom, invited us for afternoon tea in Pinzolo where he and his friends who had lived in the UK and the USA met daily, spoke English and remembered the good times abroad. In trying to keep alive aspects of their lives abroad, many returnees have invented their own (often new) traditions. For example, as noted earlier one of the most popular summer events in Carisolo, attended indistinguishably by American and British returnees, is the 4 July celebrations.

Although, on returning, migrants had fulfilled a life-long dream, many of them experienced a sense of displacement. On returning to Sicily Maria suffered from what she saw as a lack of recognition of her *sacrifici* by those who had not emigrated. This was a theme that emerged in several interviews of returnees. They felt that increased economic stability in Italy (especially in the north) had meant that local people had forgotten about poverty and the crucial contribution of those who had emigrated, left jobs and properties to those who stayed behind, and sent vital remittances. Many returnees were also disappointed by the lack of cooperation and support they received from fellow townspeople in Italy. They subsequently felt that friendship networks were stronger in Britain than in Italy and missed the solidarity they experienced in difficult times in Britain. Gianna (interviewed in Trentino, August 2005) felt that because in Trentino 'everybody is rich', people were not interested in the returnees nor in giving something back to them. For her 'everybody is just interested in themselves and in making money'. Having returned in search of strong community ties, some realized that those were stronger abroad.

Returnees found themselves having to adjust to a new situation they had not anticipated. They had hoped to retire to a place that was familiar to them, where they knew everyone and their behaviour was understood. However, they now found themselves having to cope with changes on different scales. On the one hand, the villages they left had undergone dramatic cultural, social and economic change. On the other hand, in addition to these external changes, the returnees had also changed as a result of living and working in another country for many years. Rather than simply 'fitting in', as they had hoped, they still felt somehow different from those around them and had to learn how to live their lives in places that were at once both more traditional than, and also as modern and atomized as, the society in Britain they had wished to escape.

For Riberesi a major problem caused by return was economic insecurity. They compared their present difficulties in making ends meet with their time in the UK where each couple could have two regular salaries that allowed them to live comfortably. Upon return women became full-time housewives whereas men went back to the unpredictability of agricultural work. Tina poignantly expressed the problem, when she told us that she 'liked the UK very much and if you asked around I guarantee that you would get the same answer from everybody. There we had jobs and we had no worries, life was easier' (Tina, interview location: Ribera, June 2005).

Contrary, therefore, to what migrants may think, return can mean a loss of social capital, a loss of resources and possibilities of socialization, and a loss of cooperation outside the family. They may have to come to terms with not being an ethnic minority any longer, losing the solidarity and support that sometimes had developed as a response to the exclusion that migrants faced, especially in the early migration years.

Experiencing return: migrants' offspring

With regard to the experiences of migrants' offspring who decide to 'return' to their parents' homelands, there were differences as well as similarities among those of Italian and Caribbean backgrounds. One major difference between them appeared to have been the opportunities for upward social and economic mobility.

The 'return' experience for Caribbean returnees appeared to have been economically successful. They felt that in the Caribbean they were in a better position than in Britain to utilize their British skills and qualifications to set up their own businesses and develop their entrepreneurial potential. For example, the Jamaican tourist costal towns provided young adults with ideal sites to set up their businesses. They could use their English accent to speak and relate to the many English and US tourists who took holidays in these areas. Having an English accent created particular advantages for them by making it easier than for many of those who had not migrated to apply for and securing business loans. Others were able to utilize their English accent to apply for work, without having formal or appropriate levels of qualifications. This was particularly the case in the hotel and catering industry, where some returnees acknowledged that having an English accent alone could secure a receptionist/front-of-house post, because of the common perception in these countries as well as among foreign business people that an English accent established a professional atmosphere and would attract other English and foreign customers to the place of business.

Potter and Phillips' study (2006) of migrants' offspring 'returning' to Barbados explored the power of the English accent and its symbolic associations to whiteness in postcolonial discourses. As in Jamaica, their respondents in Barbados reported similar experiences of social and economic privilege on account of their English accent and the way in which they accrued a 'pseudo-white identity' in the workplace and other professional settings that translated into power and racialized privilege over native-born black residents. Potter and Phillips pointed to the 'hybrid' or 'in-between' status of these Bajan-British 'returnees' on account of their symbolic whiteness. The returnees in our study recognize that their English accent firmly re-establishes their 'insider/outsider' status, which was earlier attributed to them as UK nationals living in Britain on account of their subordinated racial identity.

Having an English accent and an 'insider/outsider' status in these instances was utilized as an important social capital resource in generating economic opportunities for these migrants' offspring. For many of the respondents who were working and living in tourist towns, the cosmopolitan feel to the area (such as regular contact with foreign-born nationals and tourists, supermarkets that sold English and foreign goods), provided them with a strong (though probably false) sense of security, safety and familiarity, reaffirming their 'insider status'. Yet, they recognized that outside of these specific contexts and in the perceptions of the local residents they were regarded, and indeed identified themselves, as 'outsiders'. The respondents' strong networks and ties to family members in the parents' homeland celebrated their 'insider' statuses as a result of family belonging and communal bonds, whilst simultaneously highlighting their 'outsider' status on account of the obvious cultural differences between themselves and their local-born family members.

All the migrants' offspring whom we interviewed were aware that they were considered as 'outsiders' by local residents. Indeed, these interviewees 'returned' with the expectation that they would be perceived in this manner. This directly contrasts with the experiences of many older returnees who returned 'home' with the expectation that they would be fully accepted by the homeland residents and integrated back into their communities. As in our Italian case described earlier, returnees subsequently encountered feelings of loss, trauma and rejection (Goulbourne 2002). This was not experienced by the migrants' children who took the decision to migrate to their parents' homeland. Freed from the burden of looking for social acceptance, the migrants' children were more able to adapt to the cultural and social changes required to settle. They developed survival strategies to compensate for their 'outsider' position in society, including seeking out friendship and developing support networks with others like themselves. Perhaps more importantly, they maintained frequent contacts with Britain, including visits in order to maintain the social support provided by their families and friends across the Atlantic. In Barbados, Patricia told us how she managed this:

> My sister lives in Tottenham [London, UK], and we're in contact every day. If we're not on the phone then we're IMing each other. Fortunately my business means I'm coming back every six months, so I still keep up with all my friends there and I don't feel like I'm missing out and it's so easy to send a quick email or IM just to say 'hi what's up?'. I'm always persuading my sister, brother and my best friends to come out and visit me … and they do so, someone is here every summer. I have quite a network of people to call on when I need it.
>
> (Patricia, interview location: Barbados, June 2003)

However, despite their creative and pragmatic approach, the young people still found themselves frustrated by their 'outsider' status and the steep learning curve they experienced in adjusting to local customs, practices and mores. The most common frustrations were expressed in terms of adapting to the slower pace of life, the poor level of customer services in shops and businesses, living with electrical power cuts, and their lack of familiarity with the many unspoken rules and customs that are a part of daily life. In Jamaica, Sandra was particularly perplexed by the habits of drivers and the road 'codes'; she told us that

> Driving is one example where I've had problems. I had to literally re-learn how to drive. Everyone ignores the speed limit signs. Everyone overtakes even on narrowest country road. People get vex [upset] if you don't move over quickly enough. People flash their car lights to signal they're going to overtake you … There's another type of flashing which means something else completely and I never remember which is which! No-one knows where these rules come from.
>
> (Sandra, interview location: Jamaica, August 2007)

Of course, this is not an uncommon experience for the tourist or the traveller, but can be particularly frustrating for the 'returnee' who may not in fact be a returnee and has to cope with the rough and tumble of daily life in a place they are presumed to know about. Sandra's experience therefore chimes with the experiences of Italian returnees as well as with many other observations of the 'returnee' in the Caribbean (see, for example, Plaza 2000; Potter *et al.* 2005).

There appear to be fewer economic prospects for young people 'returning' to their parents' homeland in Italy than for British young people with Caribbean backgrounds. On the whole, offspring of Italian migrants in Britain tended to have greater economic possibilities in the UK than in Italy. Contrary to the Caribbean situation, their 'foreign' status works as a disadvantage in a country where being known and having personal contacts are the keys to getting jobs and doing business. They seemed to 'return' in spite of the lack of possibilities for professional advancement. As we have seen, the reason for migrating to the parents' homeland was rarely framed in economic terms. For Italians, their UK past has been of little use. They quickly had to learn to fit in and become indistinguishable from the majority population, and so, unsurprisingly, several of our interviewees were unhappy and experienced culture shock. The majority of our interviewees of this category – mostly women – stressed the difficulties of adapting to life in Italy, and this was so irrespective of whether they went to the north or the south of the country.

For example, in Ribera Sabrina told us that when her parents decided to return she was happy, because she had liked going to Ribera on holiday, and she accepted the return as a fact. Initially it was difficult to adapt to her new school but she found good classmates who helped her, but she always wanted to go back to the UK. However, at the time of our interview, Sabrina and her husband had stable jobs (which were rare in Ribera), so it had become difficult to give up these posts and return to Britain. She was sorry for her children since she thought that they would have a better education, facilities and social life in Britain than in Ribera. Sabrina felt that the more time passed the more her English side was coming out: interestingly, as an example of this surfacing of her English side she spoke about her dislike of gossip, and how she could not stand nor get involved in women's constant talk about houses and cleaning. Like Sabrina, prompted by fond memories of holidays in Ribera, Claudia 'returned', but she later felt thoroughly disappointed with her decision. She told us that she

> thought that life in Ribera was easier. I thought I knew the place because I was coming here every year on holiday. I thought that I could enjoy the very nice property that my parents had build for us with their savings. But it's hard; I find the mentality of the town very difficult to adjust to.
>
> (Claudia, interview location: Sicily, June 2005)

This kind of disappointment was shared by others, and two of the women we interviewed actually went back to the UK after an attempt to live in Italy. For Marcella the primary reason for returning to Britain was divorce, but she felt that adjusting to Italy had proven too difficult for her. It was by going to live in Italy that Marcella realized that she was more English than she had previously thought. She felt that British-Italian and Italian are:

> [t]wo different cultures completely! I went from working for British Airways [to be completely free] to go and live in Italy in a shack with all parents in the same house, as newly-weds [and] I felt really suppressed ... as soon as I had my son, everything changed. No one would babysit. I couldn't get a babysitter [this is the early '80s okay] and 'you can't get a stranger to look after your son' I went out of my door and came down the stairs and my mother-in-law would be there ... 'He's too hot ... he's too cold ... why are you doing this? ... Why are you doing that?' And I used to answer back at the beginning because ... being English and independent. I found the Italians friendly but 'backstabbers' and when you're in Italy they always talk about you behind [your back] and I didn't really fit in although I made some very good friends who are still my friends. I hate the culture of men in bars whilst women are at home and that's what he did. He had his motorbike and Sundays it was on his motorbike.
>
> (Marcella, interview location: London, February 2004)

Moreover, living in Italy without family around can be difficult and isolating, as Marcella and Paola found. Paola told us that she

> lived in Salermo for a few years but I knew that I couldn't make a life there because the reason being was because you had to have quite a strong family to support you ... if you didn't have that then you were very much left to your own devices and I started to feel a bit like 'Oh well I just want to make something of my life' ... I don't know ... I just started to feel a bit kind of lonely, especially on Sundays and I just knew that I had to have this family thing in Italy. The family thing just became a big thing.
>
> (Paola interview location: London, March 2004)

As with all categories of 'returnees', we found that gender-related cultural expectations and practices presented challenges for the women of both groups studied.

All women returnees spoke of the loss of freedom. Activities that they took for granted in the UK could not be done in their new homelands because of cultural expectations about gender roles. Caribbean women reflected that outside of work, church-related activities, the home and other kinship contexts it was very difficult to socialize with other women in public spaces. Rum-shops and bars were exclusively masculine spaces, restaurants were for families or couples. Other social activities were also viewed according to male, female, spaces, or spaces for couples or whole families. The females remarked that, compared with their lives in England, they were much more home-centred and restricted and therefore experienced isolation and alienation because their cultural differences made it difficult to establish close friendship bonds with local female neighbours and other contacts.

Conclusion

These accounts point to the complex nature of 'return' migration, and suggest that the various categories of migrant/returnee, insider/outsider, home/away, generations, and so forth need to be analysed carefully. The experiences of 'returnees' of every kind also highlight the importance of return – not just as a practice undertook by a substantial proportion of migrants and their offspring – but as an ideal, a dream resulting in the creations of myths that sustain family identities and keep alive cross-generational links across geographical locations. The 'return' is full of unexpected consequences, and as we suggest in the concluding chapter, several aspects of current migration policies may need to be critically examined in the light of what is a dynamic and relatively new form of circular migration.

Note

1 The notion or obligation of *sacrifici* (sacrifice) punctuates narratives of migration. For example, the act of migration is itself often described as being part of the *sacrifice* for the good of the family. As with many other migrants within and outside our samples, migration is perceived to be a temporary experience, with members returning to the point of departure with greater economic security.

9 Alienation and escape from the family and community

Introduction

Most of our discussion so far has focused on the positive aspects of families and communities, highlighting their strength and resilience and describing in some detail the kind of resources they provide to their members, such as care, security and a sense of identity, well-being and belongingness. In this chapter, we want to focus instead on the less positive side of families and communities, paying attention to such factors of normal life as disharmony, tensions, and imposed restraints and constraints on family members and memberships of ethnic categories or groups. It is important to discuss these negative aspects of transnational family life, because we want to transcend the simple dichotomy that persists in much journalistic as well as social capitalogic accounts of families in minority ethnic communities, where some families are seen as 'broken' (for example, Caribbeans), oppressive (for example, Muslims or Asians); or where families and communities are seen as wholly dysfunctional or wholly supportive of members. In particular, we discuss here the tensions and conflicts, alienation, and some of the negative consequences of collective belongingness and cultural identities as these relate to transnational families and communities.

Tensions and conflicts in family relationships

Feminist and other theorists (for example, Oakely 1972; Bourdieu 1997) have long drawn attention to the power struggles that go on in families, but less attention has so far been given to the centrality of emotions for understanding families and relationships. As many feminist authors have shown (Smart and Shipman 2004; Charles *et al.* 2008) most relationships are longstanding and not as easily cancellable as may be suggested by some adherents of the individualization thesis. Most individuals are involved in ties and responsibilities that require ongoing negotiations rather than in loose relationships that can be left when they become difficult. Many individuals thus often live with difficult ongoing relationships. Smart has drawn attention to the darker side of families and the emotions they produce with regard to feelings of anxiety, hurt and lack of respect which, in her view, are common in everyday family lives. She argues that the feeling of anxiety may be particularly acute in immigrant families due to the insecurity provoked by migrants' marginal position in the receiving society. Of course, this can also go in the opposite direction as family members living in hostile social conditions harness their resources to unite against onslaughts from without. Our earlier chapters have given enough examples of this. This does not, however, mean that there are not sufficient anxieties in immigrant families to bring to the surface issues arising from problems connected to customs about shame and respectability, or to honour and shame as described in much anthropological literature (see for example, Skeggs 1997). Other feelings addressed by Smart in the context of parent–children relationships in post-divorce families, such as hurt and distress, also apply to immigrant families.

Another aspect of Smart's argument is that disrespect reflects unequal power relationships within families, which may result in weaker members being ignored, disregarded or neglected. We found this to be very relevant to an understanding of some of what some of our interviewees had to say about their family lives. Similarly, the point that emotional support in families is not without strings, resonates with our findings, despite opposite claims. As Charles *et al.* (2008) asserted, support can be used to shape behaviour.

In addition to these factors is the feeling of guilt, that is, the feeling of having gone against perceived norms and obligations within families and communities. As Shaha (2007: 36) has argued: 'There are multiple arenas of contention within immigrant families and these might not necessarily engender relationships characterised by trust, cooperation and mutual obligation.'

But, as we have seen in previous chapters, such networks appear generally to be the source of much help and support to family members. We must, however, recognize that these very same resources can be mobilized to have a much darker side. As with sociological literature on the family, a critique that has been moved to the social capital literature is that it tends to emphasize the positive sides of strong networks, idealize the cooperative nature of some ethnic groups and in so doing can overlook power relations within families, communities and groups (Portes 1998; Molyneaux 2001; Zontini 2004b).

In the remainder of this chapter we illustrate some of these points from our research with families and communities in Britain, the Caribbean and Italy. We organize our comments, first, around the question of alienation experienced within families and communities drawing mainly on our Italian example; and, second, using the Caribbean example we discuss aspects of what our Caribbean respondents saw as the negative consequences of belongingness and cultural identity.

Alienation in families and communities

Many of the negative feelings reported to us originated from families struggling to cling to particular family practices and expectations, and some of these practices involved gender and generational divisions, family togetherness, and norms and values. Dissatisfaction around the gendered division of work inside and outside the household also involved issues of freedom and control for individuals. Marta recalled how she divorced her husband because he was expecting her to do everything. She explains:

Well his mum used to wash his back and put his clothes on his bed that he was going to be wearing that night and they were served hand and foot in this family, you know, I should have known then, I should have seen it, but I said to Gino you know I'm not like your mother, I said, you know I'm not like an Italian woman, I'm not going to serve you! He expected me to be his mother. He wouldn't do anything, nothing at all, at all.

(Marta, interview location: London)

It should be noted here that Marta interpreted as 'un-Italian' the desire for a fairer division of domestic work. She did not put up with her unhappy marriage and left her husband, but this was not without consequences. Her family did not approve of her decision, which they thought would bring shame on their family. Given that it was Marta who initiated the divorce and that her reasons for doing so were seen by others as well as herself as her refusal to be 'a proper Italian woman' her own mother sided with her son-in-law rather than with her daughter. Eventually, Marta was forced out of the flat in her parent's house, while her ex-husband continued to live there.

Of course, this situation is not entirely unknown in other family situations across cultures. For example, some Caribbean women also expressed resentment towards parental control or the uneven distribution of domestic tasks in the household. Many of the Caribbean young women we interviewed told us that their mothers expected them to provide the bulk of domestic support in the home from a very young age. But their mothers did not have similar expectations of their sons. This became a primary source of tension between many brothers and sisters, which continued long into adulthood. Christina in London clearly explained this situation in her own family, thus:

I know for a fact that lots of Caribbean families are run by lone mothers so effectively if they have any male children then any son becomes the man of the house. But do they really do anything? Look at my little brother, he's a classic example. He's so lazy, but it's mum's fault, she lets him get away with doing nothing. Basically she treats him like a king. But with me, now that's a different matter! When I was about seven she started showing me how to do little things around the house to help her out. When I started secondary school I was cooking, cleaning, ironing and helping with the market shopping on Saturday morning. I knew how to run a house and since then I've always been expected to help mum around the house. Whereas, my brother, well that's another story, I doubt if he even knows how to boil an egg! When I complain to mum, she just says 'oh stop complaining, oh leave my baby, he'll learn someday when he's ready and besides he's busy with college work'. But I have my work to do too and I'm still expected to help out. It's just so unfair and I've always resented my brother his easy life. He doesn't have to do anything to win mum's approval or respect. He can do no wrong in her eyes and it's always been like that. Lots of my girl-friends they say exactly the same thing because it's the same dynamic with mothers and sons. You know that saying 'mothers raise their daughters and spoilt their sons' I think that's really true. There is a whole generation of black single-mothers bringing up spoilt lazy sons, because they know that their daughters will be the ones to support them in times of need.

(Christina, interview location: London, May 2004)

Similarly, Marjorie, the eldest of five siblings and the only daughter, narrated the tension that existed between her male siblings and herself because she was expected to oversee and provide the bulk of care for their elderly parents in Guyana. This was so despite the fact that one of her brothers was living in Guyana and the other brothers in Canada and the USA lived in far closer geographical proximity to their parents than did Marjorie, who lived in London. Her story reveals the burden she carried for the family:

As the eldest and the only girl children it has always fallen on my shoulders to look after my parents. It's getting to be a bit of a burden because I'm not get-ting any younger and they're getting older and weaker too and they need more attention. But it's not shared equally [with brothers]. I have to carry the burden on my own. Everyone expects that as the only girl child it's my duty to do this and my brothers don't really help me so much. Plus I'm the oldest so I've always looked after everyone in the family.
      Do your brothers help out at all?
A: I'm tired, fed-up and frustrated with the lot of them because they make little effort. They never show any initiative and just sit down and wait for me to tell them what to do. But why should I have to tell them all the time? They might send money occasionally but it's mostly if I asked them to cover a medical bill. But that's all they do. It's not good enough. It's me who has to fly back and forth to check on them, and see the house is properly maintained and I'm expected to go. I wish I had another sister because she could help share my load. When I complain to my brothers and ask them to help me more, they say that I'm moaning and miserable, and they stop talking to me if I complain too much but they don't understand. Sometimes my [blood] pressure goes up if I worry about it too much, so I don't take them on and I just get on with what needs to be done and do the best I can. But I really worry ... if I die before my parents then who will look after them? I can't depend on none of my brothers, they're not interested and my parents don't expect much from them either.

(Marjorie, interview location: London November 2003)

Many respondents (mostly young women) felt that their families' protection and support was often a double-edge sword. Women talked about strong emotional bonds of dependency that, in their view, were at times abused by some family members. Marta, too, like some other Italian interviewees, described this situation as 'emotional blackmail', and she gave an apt illustration, when she said that:

And I remember I phoned my mum once, from Italy, to see how everything was, and she talked to me and she said: 'oh your dad's ill' (my dad was never ill you know) 'and it's all your fault'. I was like 'oh thank you!' ... Emotional blackmail was terrible, and because my brother died in India and then my other brother went to America at the same time, I couldn't do anything. She would say, 'oh if you go I'll be all on my own' and 'you don't care if I die'. When she died, it's a horrible thing to say, but I felt relief, I felt so free, so free.

(Marta, interview location: London, December 2003)

Obviously, there were important issues of norms and values involved in such circumstances and, as noted in earlier chapters, interviewees were keen to tell us about how support is linked to the fact that the receiver is expected to subscribe to these shared values. Another interviewee, Laura, felt that those giving support wanted to influence the choices of those receiving it and that support was linked to obligations. In her view the close-knit network of people with strong reciprocal bonds and obligations that form her close family could be burdensome and a basis for interference. She compared her own Italian and her husband's English families, in the following manner:

With family members you have a relationship more ... there is more history there ... therefore it's more dense and more tense, isn't it? Whereas with my husband's family, also because of their character, the relationship is much more smooth, relaxed, friendlier, therefore altogether also nicer, because it's not burdensome and at the same time it's pleasant because you meet when you meet and you spend nice days together. Even if we discuss family things, personal things, maybe because they are English, they don't interfere, because they think it's none of their business, whereas my family, because of the histories that there are, they have to say what they think even if nobody has asked them to.

(Laura, interview location: London, February 2004)

Another interviewee, Gabriella, told us that it was this kind of interference hinted at by Laura which caused her never to rely on family when she needed support. For her to accept family support would involve her subscribing to her father's values, which she rejected. Consequently, Gabriella felt envious of the kind of unconditional support she assumed existed in non-Italian families.

The ideal of family togetherness, unity and cooperation were similarly brought into question by many young people – particularly women – who felt neglected when they were children. As with the children Parreñas (2005) studied, some of our respondents from both Italian and Caribbean backgrounds related stories about the inadequacy of care they received from their families. What is of particular significance is that in both Italian and Caribbean families interviewees spoke about the lack of care from their mothers but rarely blamed their fathers, even where fathers were involved in parenting. Parrenas explains this in the context of gender boundaries: fathers, she argued, were expected to be providers whereas mothers were expected primarily to be nurturers, and children, she argued, were reluctant to accept border crossings of respective parental roles. Extending this perspective to Caribbean families, it should be remembered that mothers are generally over-loaded with the responsibility for bringing up children, and in relative terms many fathers either excuse themselves or are excused from directly participating in parenting. Such fathers would not, therefore, necessarily feature in the reckoning of parenthood.

Another issue that is recurrent in the narratives of young British-Italian women was the burden they felt they carried by having to look after themselves from a very early age. Respondents spoke about returning home from school to empty homes, having to cook their own meals and sometimes their father's also; they had therefore to take up part of their mother's share of housework while brothers and fathers were exempt from these tasks. Naturally, many interviewees resented these early responsibilities and independence that was forced upon them (see, Parrenas 2005). As Donatella told us,

> [I] always remember feeling pretty denied as a child. I remember thinking, you know, that all the other kids were doing stuff that we weren't allowed to do, so the British kids could go out and play outside whereas we couldn't. And I don't think that was just 'cos of mum and dad, I think it was because they were Italian, they didn't trust outside. … maybe that's because mum and dad worked a lot so, you know, we would get home before them, we would let ourselves in, we would sort ourselves out, and other kids' parents would be at home, so I remember, you know, going to other people's houses for a couple of hours before going to ours. Those are the kinds of things I remember.
> (Donatella, interview location: London, March 2004)

Of course, these narratives and the feelings they express must be understood within the context of their parents' experiences as low-paid workers in a little-known and perhaps less than hospitable if not entirely hostile environment. In addition, trying to make ends meet, particularly during the early years of entry and settlement, sometimes made for a difficult family environment. In such situations, parents naturally fell back on known and tried family practices, such as strict gender and generational norms and values, and thereby sometimes exacerbating conflicts with their children (see, Shaha 2007).

Although some problems were caused by adherence to so called 'traditional' family values, many of the emotional problems described to us had a different cause, namely, the mismatch between the ideal family and the reality of everyday family life. In Italian families feelings of hurt were often the result of expectations about the ideals of familyhood not being fulfilled. Feelings of rupture caused by unmet expectations that Edwards and Gillies (2005) found among working-class families were also borne out in what many Italian families told us. The case of Donatella's family is particularly interesting in this context because it shows how different values that underpinned the idealized Italian family can actually clash against each other. Individuals are often not clear about what they should do because obligations are pervasive and implicit (rather than explicit), resulting in individual family members having different and therefore sometimes conflicting expectations of their duties. Donatella's married sister lived in Italy near where their parents had decided to retire to from Britain; the sister expected that since their parents were retired they would look after her children while she went to work. The parents, however, believed that it was the younger generation that had the duty to support the older generation, so when they retired after years of hard work in London the parents were shocked to discover that one of their daughters expected them to look after her young children. According to Donatella this clash of expectations brought many conflicts into her family, which remained unresolved. This is how Donatella described the family situation:

> They found it difficult to suddenly, not just be ... normal adults. All of a sudden in Italy one is expected to be a proper grandparent where you babysit. You know, my mum, this is not in their life plan they're there to retire. All of a sudden they found themselves in control, in charge of, you know, two children, one a baby, and it just ... they found that really, really hard. And it causes numerous arguments with my sister, it's really kind of crashed their relationship .... Well mum and dad have a very strong philosophy and they always remind us that, you know, that children are meant to look after them. They always remind us that: 'we're old now. And I don't know why your sister is doing this, why we have to look after the children. We're old now, she should be looking after us.' So by the virtue of that she insinuated that that's what she believes in terms of lifespan.
>
> (Donatella, interview location: London)

Donatella's sister relied on the value or principle of family cooperation, and assumed that her parents would give her unconditional help while she worked (as many other Italian grandparents interviewed did). The sister's expectations however contrasted with her parents' understanding of the principle of strong inter-generational relationships – for them, this meant that older people should be looked after by their children. These, perhaps legitimate, misunderstandings were hurtful to all concerned.

Another typical example of unfulfilled expectations characterized the experience of several migrant workers which emerged particularly from our fieldwork in Sicily. This was the failure to achieve family togetherness despite the *sacrifici* undertaken to this end. As noted in the last chapter, the principle of *sacrifici* compelled many young British-Italian people, particularly women, to live close to their parents, and many who had done so at times expressed regret for not having fulfilled their own personal ambitions (such as going away to study or work). Those who had taken the difficult decision to move away from the family lived with the constant feeling of guilt, leading Gabriella to confess that 'for years I just went around feeling guilty about being happy'.

The main frustrated or unfulfilled expectation in inter-generational relations was that of caring for the elderly. What summarized the experiences of most of

our interviewees is again the issue of guilt. For migrants this was the guilt of having left the home of origin and therefore not being able to be near ageing parents
and carry out their duties. For the offspring of these Italian migrants, the guilt
arose from their perception that they had failed their parents in their expectations
that they would be looked after in old age in their own homes. Rita's story is an
illustration of the point:

> But I still ... which is wrong ... I still feel guilty about putting him in the
> home ... I wish I'd been young enough and strong enough to have been able
> to lift and [so] keep him here because taking him away from his family, he
> went downhill very quickly. ... at the time the guilt is very, very high and then
> afterwards after its all settled down you also feel very guilty. Very guilty! And
> we were brought up that you never did any of this and you always kept the
> family and did your best.
>
> (Rita, interview location: London, November 2003)

The accounts illustrate Shaha's (2007) argument that strong ethnic ties might not
translate as capital, as social capital theorists seem to suggest, and family solidarity
might be a source of alienation or pressure to conform to the perceived norms of a
community. Our own work suggests that strong control and pressure to adhere to
strict norms may become the flip side of family and ethnic solidarity. This emerged
as particularly acute in the large close-knit Italian communities of post-war migration of the industrial towns of Bedford and Peterborough. Francesca, interviewed
when in her early thirties, had much to say about the role of the 'community' in
her native English town. She had to struggle to have an education since girls were
expected to help around the house and then to marry and settle in the local community. Her biggest fight was to convince her parents to allow her to go to university
in London. She eventually succeeded, but her parents (especially her father) were
never supportive of her choice, which they saw as putting them in a bad light in
the eyes of their community, because an unmarried woman living alone in a big
city was seen to be of dubious morality. Her story illustrated something of the
limits and the pressures that close-knit community and family bonds can impose
upon the individual:

> I was very interested in books and the community is very old fashioned and
> very narrow minded. They absolutely replicated the 1950s' mentality and tried
> to bring up their children in the only way they knew which was very Catholic
> and very old-fashioned and narrow. They didn't value education unlike other
> immigrant communities, they didn't value education and they certainly didn't
> value it for me as a daughter. Not just my parents, I mean the community ...
> the aspirations within the community is that you would just get married as
> quickly as possible within the community ...
>
> And for me books were my kind of salvation really and I was drawing and
> doing poetry but books particularly. ... It was very difficult. My mother was
> quite supportive, my father not at all. ... He left school when he was nine and he

had no idea ... he equated reading with being lazy so I had huge arguments and I should go and help my mother in the kitchen rather than sit around reading. I know this is very much linked with the class ... he wasn't very literate himself and there weren't any books in my house until I brought them in so ...

I think it was quite hard for my parents to come to terms with me to have quite different aspirations and that I wasn't interested in being married or going out with the local Italian who was deemed a good catch so. ... My mother was quietly supportive and then quite actively so when I decided I wanted to go to university. It was very hard for them, very hard because as I said, the community is very old fashioned so my parents really suffered ... because my brother and I left at the same time to go to university and they were left there having to deal with people's prejudices and ignorance and it was very hard. ...

They thought my father's masculinity had been tainted or damaged and they thought that I should never be allowed back home. It was very 1950s and very old fashioned and previously you see. Because my mother was a dressmaker for the community I was the perfect daughter and I spoke perfect Italian and I would read their letters for them ... so I went from having quite a particular role within the community and then to leave home was transgressing everything. God, it was very difficult in the beginning. I remember some of them when I went back to visit, they would cross the road and pretend not to see me and very prejudiced and very old fashioned about ... so leaving home was like going to be a prostitute ...

London is different ... people move in and moved around ... and they don't have the pressure of that stability of what the community was in the way that I did.

(Francesca, interview location: London, December 2003)

The story of Francesca shows that, as many feminist scholars have pointed out, escaping families and communities is not as easy as some proponents of the individualization theory sometimes appear to suggest. Individuals are closely embedded in complex networks where solidarity, responsibility and commitment are believed in, even if not always operationalized. This does not mean that our respondents had no agency and passively accepted and endured the difficult relationships they told us about. In the case of Francesca her escape was through education. Some women tried to escape from families and communities' control through 'return' migration, although sometimes with limited results, as discussed in the last chapter. While some managed to break away from unsatisfactory relationships with their parents, it appeared more difficult to make such escapes from partners.

The negative consequences of collective belonging and cultural identity

In the context of Caribbean families much of the alienation experienced in families and communities was expressed in terms of ethnic identity formation and the ways in which individuals choose to define themselves. Relationships with family and friends helped to shape the processes of ethnic identity formation for the Caribbean migrants and their offspring. The effects of these relationships were double-edged. On the one hand, new relationships were established to assert a new collective identity described as Caribbean – it must be borne in mind that before large-scale migration across the Atlantic there was little consciousness of a Caribbean-wide identity (see, Goulbourne 2008, 2002). On the other hand, in order to conform to group norms and live up to cultural expectations of a Caribbean identity it sometimes resulted in individuals valuing identities that were narrow and limited in scope. It also placed limitations on the ways in which these individuals saw themselves in terms of ethnic identity and restricted the types of activities they undertook.

For example, many of the younger Caribbean respondents whom we interviewed expressed anxiety about behaving and representing themselves in ways that went against assumed group norms and cultural practices they considered to be central to black/Caribbean racial-ethnic identity. They were particularly fearful that such activities and behaviour would lead them to be ostracized and alienated by their peers within the community, and the related pain of not belonging or being excluded if they did not conform to these assumed culturally accepted practices. Those young people who did not conform to these expected cultural practices were commonly labelled as 'acting white', which was not something these respondents wanted to be accused of by their peers and community members. Our conversation with Carol in Nottingham illustrates this problem:

Q: What types of music do you like and listen to?

A: I like all types of music; I'm a real fan of all types of music. I like the usual

Q: What's the usual?

A: Black music, you know, soul, reggae, house but I also like country and western, and classical. When I'm at home I listen to a lot of classical music … my grandparents loved classical music and I grew up listening to it and developed a passion for it. But I only listen to that at home. Never when I'm out [of house] I stick to the usual

Q: Why don't you listen to classical music when you're not at home?

A: Are you mad? I don't want my friends to 'cuss' me and I certainly don't want them to laugh at me. If they knew I was into that classical music, they would cuss me and say 'why are you listening to that posh music for? Are you acting white and pretending to be something that you are not?'.

Q: Do you believe that?

A: No but it's easier to go with the flow, my grandparents love classical music and they're Bajan (Barbadian), so it's not really music for white people. Classical music is music to be appreciated by all people. But I don't know it's what black people do isn't it? We're expected to act in a certain way. Young people have to act a certain way and only like certain things. We're expected to listen to the usual soul, rap and if you like anything different then you run the risk of being called 'whitey' or 'too white' or people will think you're just plain weird.

(Carol, interview location: Nottingham, April 2004)

In our interviews with the Caribbean young people the term 'acting white' was often repeated in their accounts, and as the discussion with Carol indicates, this was usually framed around the concern that any behaviour and activities that did not conform to, or embody the characteristics, of black youth cultural identity would be negatively viewed by others in the Caribbean community. This notion of 'acting white' is typically discussed in the arena of educational policy and linked to academic underachievement of black youth and the cultural devaluation of educational attainment among these youths.[1] Our older Caribbean respondents in both the UK and Caribbean expressed increasing concern about the way in which Caribbean young people were engaging with this discourse of 'acting white' whereby education is devalued and street culture/popular culture, which is perceived as black identity, celebrated as being both revolutionary and oppositional. Even among professional upper middle-class families in the Caribbean, many parents were anxious that their children, male children in particular, were turning away from university and the value of higher education because this was regarded by these young men as representative of a white/European/colonial model and the maintenance of the status quo (see, Chevannes 1996, 2002). Instead, an increasing number of young men from professional and upper middle-classes backgrounds expressed interest in pursuing careers in the music and entertainment industry. These industries were celebrated and valorized among the youths as representing revolutionary black culture and identity. Tension and conflict developed between these parents and their offspring over their children's aspirations because it radically departed from their own middle-class aspirations and ideals. William, who lived in Jamaica and had family members in the UK, commented thus:

> Mona University [The University of West Indies, Mona, Jamaica] is now female-dominated. I believe more women are graduating than men. The male students are dropping out. They all want to be dancehall DJs and artists. They are no longer interested in following the professional routes to success. My son is now deciding what he wants to do when he leaves school and the silly boy said that he's not certain that he wants to go to university. I find it all very distressing because he's a bright boy and we've given him every opportunity. The silly boy wants to be a music promoter, like every other boy on the island. Everyone wants to be the next Sizzla or Bounty Killa [popular reggae artists]. No one wants to be a doctor, lawyer or accountant any longer. You know what my son told me when I told him to think about those professions, he said 'Dad that's so old-fashioned and boring …. 'I said 'I'm an accountant, what is so wrong with that? It paid for the nice house you live in, your nice clothes and your good education.' But all he goes is 'Dad times have changed, that was fine for your time but my time is now and I don't want to follow the white man and be a suit and tie man and besides why waste time at university studying all those years, when I can make money now?' Can you believe the stupidity of my son! At the moment we can't get along. We're fighting everyday because I can't understand that mentality. The mentality of the young men today is so confusing. We were raised to value education and hard work. It used to be the

poorer kids who used music as a way out of poverty and to better themselves, that I can understand. But today it's also the rich kids, those who come from good backgrounds and who go to the top school in the country who also want to follow the music route. They think it's the easy route but they are so wrong because so few artists make it to the top and earn a decent living from it, but they fail to understand that.

(William, interview location: Jamaica, August 2004)

In the UK context, one explanation put forward for the narrow, essentialized and reductionist construction of black cultural identity is that black people have had to develop protective devices to promote and sustain boundaries between themselves and white dominant culture (Brah 1996; Sewell 1997). There is also an alternative perspective that suggests the notion of black cultural identity holds only negative connotations related to underachievement and limited success. The leap has not, however, been made to suggest that for Caribbean youths in Britain to achieve educational success and social mobility they must 'distance' themselves from black cultural identity and assume a 'white' or 'raceless' persona, as has been discussed in the USA (see, for example, Fordham and Ogbu 1986).

In our interviewees with the Caribbean migrants in the UK, we came across a small minority of middle-class parents who partly supported this viewpoint. For instance these respondents believed that their children becoming friends with white middle-class children would be beneficial to their children in later life and as a result they actively encouraged their children to pursue such networks.

Most of my friends are white and middle class. They [parents] encouraged me to … have friends that are successful at things, and whose parents are success-ful. So I think they were definitely strategic in some of the things they did. They moved to put my sister and me in a better school, so we could develop more successful friends.

(Anthony, interview location: London, November 2003)

There was also a small minority of parents who wanted their children to distance themselves from other black children because they feared such friendships would lead to their children being negatively stereotyped on the basis of their black racial identity. This sometimes caused their children to become uncertain about their own identities and created tensions in the parent–child relationship. The fol-lowing statement by Dominique, for example, highlights some of the tension she experienced with her mother because of the negative way in which the mother viewed black people:

It was common for my mother to say to me 'be careful not to have too many black friends because the white teachers will put you all together and assume all sorts of bad things about you, which are not true'. She always said 'If you want to make it in this world then you have to be different and not follow the crowd [of black girls].' So of course, I believed that, I never questioned it and

I tried not to move with a black crowd at school and I would only make friends with the white girls. I was confused about my own identity for years because she [mother] made me believe that being black was a bad thing, so I didn't have any black friends and I would try to pretend that I'm not black. So if someone said a racist comment I'd deny they were talking about me. I was in serious denial for years. Of course, the black girls they all hated me too because I used to ignore them and they called me 'coconut'. But I really believed that if I acknowledged I was black then I thought no one would take me seriously. I was very unhappy because of course I wasn't white and they'd [white friends] say 'Dominique, why you pretending to be white', and a part of me hated them for saying that but I hated myself more. It was a confusing time in my life. I felt that I was living a pretence and pretending to be somebody else I was not by not acknowledge my black identity.

Q: how do you feel about it now?

A: I know it's nonsense … it has damaged my relationship with her [mother], we're fine but I'm not sure we can ever repair things completely. She's got this warped view about her own people. In a way, she was saying that she doesn't respect me or think I'm worthy because I'm black, also that she doesn't value herself too, why give that message to your own child?

(Dominique, interview location: Manchester, February 2004)

There were other examples from our interviews illustrating how some Caribbean migrant parents encouraged their offspring to have white and/or other ethnic minority friends. Paradoxically, this was balanced with a concern about their children forgetting their cultural roots and heritage or becoming alienated from the wider Caribbean community. This tension in these parental expectations, however, may not be contradictory; it may well be that their strategies for their children's success is far more concerned with social class matters than with racial and ethnic identities, but the one does not necessarily negates the other. This interpretation was borne out by the fact that in instances where these children attended schools where they were one or a few of black/minority ethnic children, their parents would utilize additional resources to ensure that their children maintained interest in their cultural heritage such as regular family holidays in the Caribbean and sending their children to black supplementary schools.

When recollecting their childhood, many offspring who grew up in the 1970s and 1980s recollected their shared fears and concerns about being labelled as 'acting white' by other Caribbean offspring. At the same time they felt uncomfortable about being 'black' and Caribbean because of the negative connotations that were associated with this identity, such as being rioters and muggers. However, many interviewees acknowledged that in the new century there were more positive images of black racialized and Caribbean cultural images. This change in attitudes may have been due to what Philip in London observed:

It's very common today to see black people represented on TV in all walks of life. I've also noticed that there are more black people advertising products.

You even see black families on advertisements. It's progress definitely because my kids don't think that unusual. In my days as a youth the only time we were represented on TV was on the news and we were usually the lead stories as the muggers and rapists. That the only way that most white people who didn't live in the cities could relate to us but its changed a lot now.

(Phillip, interview location: London, September 2004)

The second key way in which alienation and exclusion by family and community members was expressed in the interviews was in relation to return migration by Caribbean offspring, which we discussed in the last chapter, and therefore we do not need to return to here. We may, however, note that in the region racial and ethnic identities are closely intertwined with social class. For example, status and power have historically been strongly associated with a white or European upper class. Debates exploring the intersections of race, class and gender have continued to be significant in the present century. For example, during a third visit to Jamaica for fieldwork in 2007, the country was building up to its national elections and the leaders (Bruce Golding and Portia Simpson) of the two major parties that have always formed the government were sharply divided along racial and ethnic, class and gender lines, with the one perceived to be representative of the white/brown owning classes and the other representative of the working classes, women and the intelligentsia.

One respondent spoke of the shock she experienced about the direct and overt references made in relation to people's skin colour and the way in which this positioned people's class and social interactions in Jamaican society. However, her 'outsider status' enabled her to distance herself from this racial stereotyping and herself being stereotyped. She stressed that she

was disappointed by work colleagues and their treatment of Portia Simpson [at time of national election]. People were saying 'we can't have a black woman representing us; it looks bad for the country'. Well I'm black and I assumed I was middle class, but no maybe I'm not so sure what I am. When I approached my work friend about the Portia issue she said, 'Jennifer you're different, you're English but if you were from Jamaica do you think that you as a black woman could get so far, so quickly? That's when I noticed the colour and class issue because I was the only dark-skinned woman in that senior position. Jamaica hasn't changed in that respect.

(Jennifer, interview location: Jamaica 2007)

Another respondent also used the national elections to highlight his 'foreigner status':

Portia must get in again [re-elected] because she's a woman and she's black, and they're in the majority, so she'll get the majority of support. I never realized this race thing ran so deep still but its very much part of Jamaica though we like to think that we're all one people.

Q: How do you define your class?

A: I have working-class roots but here I'm 'foreigner' and I don't know if people think of me in class terms.

(Wayne, interview location: Jamaica 2007)

These conversations indicated that while there has been considerable social change over the last half century – such as increased opportunities for upward social mobility for the majority black population – class remained intricately linked to colour and colour is still deeply ingrained in the national culture and psyche. From an early age many children learn about colour discrimination, and the family act as a major agent in transmitting these values of skin colour (see, for example, Smith 1965, 1984). Various customs, beliefs, attitudes and types of behaviour continue both explicitly and implicitly to valorize white identity whilst at the same time pathologizing black identity in a number of different ways. For example, skin bleaching is still popular amongst some dark-skinned women in order to achieve a lighter skin tone; so too, as in Britain, is the wearing of false hair (wigs and extensions) to appear like white European or brown Asian women, rather than like themselves. Skin bleaching and the wearing of false hair have led to a highly successful commercial business in these areas in the Caribbean as in Britain. One respondent who admitted to using these products shared anecdotal stories about her fears of being 'too black' and the belief that brown-skinned women (sometimes colloquially referred to as 'brownings') were favoured as partners by men over dark-skinned women. Such notions of physical beauty and desirability are by no means exclusive to any one Caribbean society; indeed, such understandings of female beauty, sexuality and desirability are common across the Caribbean and African diasporas (see, for example, Cooper 1995).

The offspring returnees recognized that in Britain their black racialized identity unified them and much of their experience was framed around this collective identity. In the Caribbean they were exposed to the hierarchal racial and class structures underpinning privilege and power among diverse groups of homeland residents. During interviews with the native-born homeland residents in the three selected Caribbean countries (Barbados, Guyana and Jamaica), sometimes there was a reluctance to explicitly acknowledge the issue of colour privilege as a significant determinant of class location and social status. The young 'returnees', in contrast, were very willing to highlight and reflect on this issue, perhaps because their 'outsider' status excluded them from being structurally positioned in this manner and because they came from a Britain where racial differentiation is a matter of public discourse. In the Caribbean, this remains a relatively shunned problem; racial matters have yet to become the public issue they are in Britain or the USA.

As with Italian migrants' offspring 'returnees', Caribbeans of the same generation spoke extensively of their loss of freedom. Activities that they took for granted in Britain could not be assumed in their new country of settlement because of the different cultural expectations established along gender lines. They reflected that outside of work, church-related activities, the home and other kinship contexts it was very difficult to socialize with other women in public spaces. For example, as noted above, rum-shops and bars were exclusively masculine spaces, restaurants family and/or couple spaces. Other social activities were also gendered. There were, of course, some differences according to urban–rural settings. In Jamaica, for example, unmarried and or single women in the capital city of Kingston had more space to socialize with their female friends (such as going to the cinema or the gym) than did women who lived in rural areas. Social spaces outside the home and work were very restricted for both married and single women in rural areas.

> If women are out with female friends without their children or family relations, [it's] assumed that you're up to no good, either you're looking for a man. ... Men get very insecure and threatened when they see a group of women out together maybe because the men are very chauvinistic here, they [men] know how they behave when they're out, so they think that it must follow that another man is trying to do that [chat-up] with their woman.
>
> (Denise, interview Jamaica, August 2007)

All female interviewees commented on culturally defined sexual dynamics as challenging. They were aware that they were living in a society where a degree of gender segregation operated. Outside family or romantic circles, men and women did not appear to interact with each other and it was difficult to establish cross-gender friendships. For example, it was difficult for women to have males as platonic friends without observers assuming that their relationship was of a sexual nature. Married women in platonic friendships with other men felt that they were criticized in their communities and families, because it was expected that these women should only socialize with husbands or male family members.

Denise's story illustrates this point. She had a platonic friendship with a male, but this led to considerable social pressures and difficulties because she was seen to be undermining acceptable notions of female behaviour and friendship patterns. When Denise married her Jamaican partner, Trevor, his sexuality was called into question for allowing her friendship to continue in such a public manner, and he faced pressure from his friends and family members to put an end to the friendship in order to assert his manhood. However, Denise was allowed to continue the friendship on account of her being 'foreign'. In this instance her 'outside' status allowed her to negotiate a gendered identity that fell outside of culturally prescribed norms.

Compared with their lives in England, the women felt their lives to be much more home-centred, and therefore experienced isolation and alienation; like our Italian interviewees in much the same situation, these women found that their British cultural baggage made it difficult to establish close friendships with the local females. In Jamaica, Beverley told us that she had

> loads of acquaintances. I know lots of people that I've met now in church, and stuff like that. Friends? I don't have many ... I'm different. We just think differently, and I have a problem communicating with them on a genuine level.
>
> (Beverley, interview location: Jamaica, August 2007)

Sandra told us much the same story, when she said

> Yeah, I have some people I'm friendly with but I don't really have them as close friends here, because I have a serious problem with them. We're just … we're not … we don't think alike. I'm too open, and because of that, you're subject to all sorts of … abuse and liberty taking. They can't help it! When I used to open my home and invite the friends, you know, they'd just come, and, you know, at first it was cool, you know but then they just started to come whether they're invited or not. They'd come, and they eat out your food. You know, they don't contribute anything. In England, you just bring something, you know, just to put back. But here, they don't have that concept, you know. It's food, it's free. They've got nothing to put back.
>
> (Sandra, interview location: Jamaica, August 2007)

Sexual jealousies also appeared to have played a part in these women's isolation. Enjoying the status of being 'foreign' and possessing an 'English accent' were seen to endow special privileges for the women from England which made it easier for them to attract men. In such instances it could be suggested that having what is thought to be an 'English accent' represented an important social resource for British women of Caribbean backgrounds in subverting cultural notions of beauty and desirability, which were conventionally defined around skin colour. Georgia was very aware of this as part of Jamaica's social environment, when she told us that

> It's very competitive here, that's why you see so many well groomed women. They may have spent their last pay cheque getting the hair, nails and clothes just perfect and have no food to live on for the rest of the week. But the mentality here is that women dress up and always look sexually desirable, always there's no let up and I find that really frustrating. Sometimes I run to the corner shop with my old shorts and jeans on but I know if I'm seen out like that people will talk about me and what I wearing, when I say people I mean the women because they are very judgemental and always in each other business. … I miss my old life in London where I am completely anonymous and there's not this pressure to look good all the time …. Being English you're definitely more at an advantage though because you don't have to be the prettiest or [wearing] expensive designer clothes because your accent alone can carry you through. The men love the English accent. English women stand out from the crowd and we are different to the Jamaican they are used to. The women can't stand it because they may be really pretty but they can never get the accent and they hate it!
>
> (Georgia, interview location: Jamaica, August 2004)

It was therefore to the advantage of these women to develop new ways of negotiating their way into the society by maintaining elements of their British gender identity.

Men of the same backgrounds did not experience the same reception. Part of this could be attributed to the different ways in which male and female friendship bonds are generally formed. For example, it would appear that where intimate emotional bonds are significant in forming female friendships and there is value in 'being there' for each other, male friendships may be more dependent on social and recreational factors (see, for example, Allan and Adams 1999; Pahl 2000; Pahl and Pevalin 2005; Reynolds 2007).

The men regarded their friendship ties to have been formed in more instrumental ways, and because they did not depend upon these male friendship bonds for intimacy and emotional support they were able to establish friendship networks with the local men relatively quickly. However, it should also be noted that the men's freedom of movement in public spaces also facilitated their ease in adjusting. Their ability to negotiate public spaces and participate in many aspects of social life meant that they did not experience as many problems as the female returnees. This in turn allowed them to meet and establish friendly relations with local men. The rum-shops, bars, beachfronts, the cultural practice of 'liming' (hanging out on the street and engaging in verbal bantering) and their participation in sporting clubs such as the local football and cricket teams all facilitated social contact and integration. Being 'English' or the 'English boy' marked them as 'different' or as 'outsiders', and this sometimes made them the brunt of jokes and friendly banter, but this identification did not create difficulties because being 'foreign', particularly British or American, can be a social advantage.

Although not as vitally important as with British Italians settling in the land of their parents, personal contacts and family bonds were important in the project of entry and settlement for such everyday matters as childcare as well as finding employment or developing business opportunities. In most cases, the family networks provided components of social capital such as, for example, care, support and reciprocal trust. However, there were other examples which showed that family networks of support sometimes broke down and relations quickly soured. Tina in Jamaica described a case whereby family members used the expectation of reciprocal support and trust to take advantage of a family member:

> My cousin lost her job but she had some financial problems. I loaned her the money and we had arrangement that she would collect the children from school and fix them a light supper until we got home from work. But she was always borrowing money and final straw was when I found out the children weren't getting anything to eat until we got home in the evening. I had to let her go but then we were faced with the problem of all the lies and malicious rumours she was spreading. It caused bad feeling in the final … and at the time I decided we needed to distance ourselves and try to get by on our own without depending on them so much. Families can be strength but they can also be a burden.
>
> (Tina, interview location: Jamaica, August 2007)

Conclusion

Participation, therefore, in strong family and ethnic networks both within and across national boundaries has both positive and negative implications for individuals. In earlier chapters we saw examples of what may be considered some positive aspects, and in this chapter we focused on aspects of the disappointments and pain, conflicts and misunderstandings brought about by broken expectations – often accompanied by feelings of guilt and regret – as well as how strong ethnic groups can preserve community cohesion and shared norms at the expense of their individual members. This may be an appropriate point at which to turn to the related matter of the crossing of boundaries.

Note

1 Harpalani (2004), partly correctly, but also partly misleadingly, argued that black identity, such as a Caribbean identity, is constructed as an oppositional cultural and racial identity to 'white identity'. This raises issues that go beyond the scope of this particular discussion.

10 Crossing boundaries

Problems and opportunities in 'mixed' families

Introduction

A key dimension of transnational family life in diverse Britain is what is increasingly being described as 'mixed' families. Of course, at the simplest level of their formations all families are naturally to one degree or other mixed, because individuals combine to start such relationships that eventually result in the complex structures and social practices we understand as families and kinship groups. In the last chapter we discussed how individual members of families and kinship networks as well as wider racial and ethnic communities do not always find fulfilment in their families, groups or communities to which they feel they belong. One way out of the impasse into which such feelings or disappointments may lead is the inauguration of social change within families and racio-ethnic groups; another is for individuals to cross harder boundaries into other communities through marriage, the production of children, sharing of households, and other forms of living arrangements. The acceptance of diversity in contemporary Britain and the emergence of transnational families are developments compelling social analysts to revisit the problematic of the processes of raciation and the construction of new ethnicities within the context of family life.

In this chapter we therefore turn attention to some problems involved in crossing important boundaries as illustrated by our respondents' narratives. More specifically, we organize the discussion around what may be regarded as intra-ethnic/ intra-racial and inter-ethnic/inter-racial, but in doing so we also bring into focus mixing across other boundaries such as that of region, and differential migration experience as illustrated by British Caribbeans and British Italians.

Intra-ethnic/racial 'mixed' families

We start with the 'invisible' boundary that separates and informs social relations between 'established' and 'newly arrived' Caribbean communities in Britain. Over half a century after the docking of SS *Empire Windrush* in Essex in 1948, we can legitimately talk about 'established' Caribbean communities as distinct from the 'newly arrived' from the region in recent decades. This new wave of migration is partly encouraged by the presence of existing Caribbean communities in major UK cities. It is assumed that the newcomers can be readily integrated into earlier communities and that this process would be facilitated by the continuing strong Caribbean transnational kinship networks.

Unfortunately, however, comparatively little research has been conducted into the lives of the newcomers, and whilst it is generally assumed that they have been comfortably inserted into the established communities, we found that there is some distance between the two groups. For example, Lloyd, who was born and brought up in Britain, found himself in an awkward situation with some newcomers who appeared to have moved into his familiar social space, the pub. Lloyd told us that

> there is a difference that no one ever talks about .... I notice within our community we're isolating ourselves more from each other. I don't think it's deliberate or intentioned but people go where they are comfortable. The pub down the road is a place we used to go there but now it's taken over by a new [migrant] group of Jamaicans. We stopped going there because it's a real hard-core Jamaican pub now
>
> Q: Hardcore? What do you mean?
> A: Hard-core as in the authentic thing, real Jamaicans from 'yard',[1] who have not too long come over [migrated to England].
> Q: Ok, and is that why you stopped going to the pub?
> A: No ... well, yeh, I guess but I don't think I ever said 'I'm not going anymore' but I just accepted that the pub is now their [newcomers] place, its where they go to chill and hang out. As a British-born black person you would have to be really confident to go in there because it's obvious you don't belong. The last time I went there I just stood out and looked out of place and sort of uncomfortable. Everyone looks like they know everyone else and they were talking about stories and news event back home [Jamaica] because they have just arrived in England and so everything happening in Jamaica is current and fresh to them. All I really know is what my parents tell me and they're a bit out of touch with what's going on in Jamaica now.
>
> (Lloyd, interview location: Birmingham, April 2004)

In London, Sherry, the daughter of an 'established' Jamaican migrant, gave her powerfully considered opinion of the 'newly arrived' migrant and outlined her perceptions of some differences between these sub-groups within her community:

> The 'just-come' Jamaicans always stand out. You'd pick them out in the crowd before they open their mouth. Its wrong to stereotype but they are a definite type. They look different to us.
>
> Q: Can you give me an example please?
> A: There's nothing specific I can point to, but you know it when you seen them. It's more to do with the way they carry themselves. They walk with more confidence and they want to stand out from the crowd. The attitude is 'don't mess with me'. Their clothes are brighter and they tend to wear more American gear: basketball hats and shirts, always designer. They always have designer gear and

they want show it off. I think they're more bold and brash, and more in your face. Everything is more bigger and brasher ... whereas we [established] tend to more conservative and take after the English in that respect but the 'just-come Jamaican' will wear all his designer items from head-to-toe, and will keep the label hanging out [of clothes] so everyone can see its Dolce and Gabbana, Moschino, Armani, Roc-A-Wear or Timberland. I think they're motto for dressing in designer gear is, 'the more the merrier', whereas we are much more subtle and will mix our clothes more and not want to show it all off at once and wear so much of it at one time. Also the accent is also pretty full-on but you would expect that if they have just come [to England].

(Sherry, interview location: London, November 2003)

Sandra in Manchester added factors of gender and class to these stereotypes when she qualified an earlier statement by saying

Don't take this the wrong way, because we're all one-blood but when you asked me the difference [with newcomers] I immediately pictured the dance-hall queen, you know what I mean, wearing skin-tight and bright clothing, false nails and elaborate hair-styles, a bit vulgar, trashy and downmarket .... I'm so sorry I shouldn't have said that and I can't think why that picture immediately came to mind. ... I know they don't really dress like that, and well only some women dress up to that extent if they're going on a night-out. ... What I really believe is that the [newcomer] women are much more confident with their looks and well they don't give a damn about being a size 0 toothpick! If they like it then they'll wear it and I've seen some big, big, big women squeezed into some tiny piece of something! They don't care. It's good that they haven't been influenced by the English ways yet and the message that says 'the skinner you are the more beautiful you are'. But black women born here we're more influenced by those ideals. I think they [newcomer] haven't been brainwashed yet.

(Sandra, interview location: Manchester, January 2004)

Sandra's was just one of many views which suggested that the new arrivants had a lower social status than those who had arrived here earlier. The social and sexual morality of the newcomers was also commented upon, but at the same time they were admired for their uniqueness, sense of individuality and their lack of conformity to British cultural norms and practices.

The 'newly arrived' migrants were likewise critical of the 'established' migrants and their offspring. For example, Murphy from Guyana pointed to what he saw as the opportunities missed by children born to Caribbeans in Britain; he noted that

the main difference is that we [newcomers] appreciate life more and work hard to take every opportunity we can get to make a better life. But the black English who grow up in this country they are so spoilt. You see the little youths running around. They walk the streets with trousers hanging down their ankles and they have a bad attitude. Honestly, its gets me so mad when I sit and think too much about it. I don't have any time or respect for them because they don't realise how good life is here [UK]. You English have it really good here, you don't know what it is to really suffer and grow up hard [with poverty and hardship]. When I first arrived I was so surprised that the kids don't want to go to school and it's free. That is madness! All the opportunities are here for them if they make a little effort but they don't appreciate it. The children in Guyana would cry out for an opportunity for free schooling, the youths in England are spoilt brats who need a reality check.

(Murphy, interview location: London, May 2004)

Similarly, Rianna from Barbados remarked that

I don't know too much about the [established] men but I do know British-Caribbean women are far too stoosh [arrogant] and unfriendly. They [established] think they are somehow better or cleverer than us [newcomers] because their parents were immigrants 50 or so years ago. But as little as our country is [Barbados] education-wise we are much more advanced and as a people much more educated. Yet we don't walk around looking down on others. We are much more tolerant. The thing that surprised me most though is that lots of Caribbean young people don't go to church. They don't have that Christian values or morals and that's why the reason this country has so many problems with the young. In our country everyone goes to church, young and old. Apart from that I would say we are more similar than different.

(Rianna, interview location: London, January 2004.)

While each group had strong views about the other, it is interesting to note that there were many couples composed of new male arrivants and females born in Britain to Caribbean migrants. These unions revealed divisions and tensions across an 'invisible' intra-ethnic boundary, and concerns were mainly expressed about issues of residency, the cultural adjustment of the new arrivant and the response of family and friends.

First, where couples from significantly different backgrounds should live was often a matter of concern to the couples themselves as well as to other members of their families. In many cases, for intra-ethnic couples the question was about whether to continue living in Britain, in the Caribbean homeland, or in Canada or the USA. It was felt by the 'newcomer' that these other countries had a broader range of opportunities and scope for social mobility compared with life in Britain. For example, Maria, the offspring of Jamaican-born parents who arrived in Britain in the early 1950s, met her husband, Dennis, in 1997 during a family holiday in Jamaica. Over the following two years Maria and Dennis would visit each other in Jamaica and England, and in 2000 they decided to get married so that Dennis could enter and settle in Britain. Although Dennis was granted full British citizenship, he found life difficult in England. A chartered surveyor in Jamaica, Dennis became concerned with finding similar employment in England.

At the time of interview Dennis could find only poorly paid construction labour work and as a result he believed that his skills and qualifications were wasted in Britain. He particularly disliked what he described as the 'mentality of English employers', that is their dismissive attitudes towards his educational qualifications gained at a elite Jamaican school and degree from the University of West Indies in Jamaica. In time, Dennis came to see this as racial discrimination, and became keen to emigrate to the USA or Canada, where his siblings and kin members lived. He was confident that in either of these countries he would have better employment opportunities and an improved chance of upward social mobility. His dream was within 10 years to make enough money to return home to Jamaica, where he planned to set up his own construction and chartered surveyor business. He envisaged that the time he would spent in North America would not only enable him to raise sufficient funds to realize his dream, but this time would also allow him to establish important networks and contacts with 'returning' Jamaicans in order to secure future construction contracts.

Dennis' dreams and plans contrasted sharply with his wife's hopes for the future. Maria was born and lived all her life in the Ladywell district of Birmingham, had strong family and friendship ties in the locality, and therefore had no desire or plan to leave. She was employed in a relatively secure (and long-term) local government job, and her two children from a previous relationship meant that she had a network of good childcare support, including the children's non-resident father, his parents, and the children's paternal grandparents. Maria was adamant that she did not want to migrate, on what she termed 'a whim' for a number of reasons. Firstly, she did not want to disrupt her children's education and family life by moving to another country; she believed that by emigrating she would loose invaluable social and care support provided by her extended kin who live close by; and she was concerned that her children's father would loose contact with his offspring. Moreover, he would use her departure as grounds to seek legal custody of the children.

Unfortunately, Maria and Dennis were unable to resolve this issue. Dennis felt that he had no 'strong pull' to England, other than his wife and the children, and he believed that his wife should support his decision to emigrate, while Maria could not jeopardize her close-knit family and neighbourhood. As Dennis was aware of this situation when he met her, she felt that he should make the commitment to their lives in England and forget his dreams and plans to emigrate. At the time of our interview, this issue was still unresolved and Dennis was planning to go to Houston, Texas, on a temporary basis to take up a construction contract for three months and also use the time 'to see what's out there and see what works out'. Dennis was resolute that if a better employment opportunity arose elsewhere then he would not remain in England, while Maria was equally determined that England was her home and under no circumstance would she leave.

Second, adapting to different cultural attitudes around gender roles caused tension and divisions among Caribbean 'established' and 'newly arrived' couples. It was commonly recognized by these couples that despite a shared cultural heritage and origin, being a 'newly arrived' or 'established' created significant differences in their partnership or marriage. The British-born women, for example, commented on the 'chauvinistic' attitude of their 'newcomer' male partners and the way in which there was a cultural expectation that, outside of work, family and child-related activities, women should remain in the private domain. These women believed that their male partners expected to police and monitor their women's activities in the public sphere, especially social activities, to a far greater degree than these women would expect from British-born men. As one female respondent, married to a newly arrived migrant noted:

> On the surface they pretend to be laid-back because that's the Jamaican thing, the men are supposed to laid-back, cool, 'no problem, man' and pretend that nothing fazes them and they must always show they're in control of their emotions …. But I've detected a big chauvinism compared to British men. Or maybe they're less sneaky about it! I don't know what it is but they have this definite mentality where its 'I'm the man so I can go out all night with my friends and I don't expect you to ask me about it.' Murphy expects me not to ask too many questions about his business because that's what he's used to but he expects to ask me about my whereabouts. When I challenge him on this usually he says 'I'm a man and we need our space sometimes without all the questions, but you're my woman so it's different'. He'll ask more questions about where I'm going? Who I'm going to be with? What time I'm coming home? etc., etc., and then there's all the phone calls pretending to see if I'm ok but really I know he's only calling to check up on me to see what I'm up to.
>
> (Amanda, interview location: Nottingham, February 2005)

Many of the women were the main economic breadwinners in the family but the men expected to exercise authority in the home, such as having the last voice in marital or partnership matters.

Another cause for concern by these women were the openly homophobic views and attitudes expressed by their newly arrived partners. Homophobic attitudes are common in many Caribbean countries, and many of these men arrive in Britain with such attitudes. An example of this concern is that of Clement, a Jamaican, who arrived in England 15 years before our interview, and his wife, Joy, who was an offspring of Caribbean migrants. Although the interview was originally with Clement, Joy arrived home from work midway through the interview and she was invited to contribute to the rest of the discussion. Part of the conversation illustrates their differing attitudes:

Q: Clement, what has been the main source of disagreement?
C: We don't have any problems, we get on fine, it's irie [good]. The one time we argue is about one of her friends dem, the *battyman*.[2] I can't understand why she wants to be friends with him.
Q: What's his name?
C: I don't know his name and I don't want to know his name. I don't want to know nothing about him.

J: [Joy shouts to Clement from the kitchen] His name is Stephen and you know that, so why are you lying? You know we're work friends and he's a good friend of mine.

C: I don't want to know, I'm not interested in your friend and who he be. One time she wanted to bring the *battyman* to the house. I said 'no way, that can happen as long as I'm living under this roof, I don't want people like that around me.'

Q: Joy, how do you feel about that?

J: It's just the way Jamaican men are, they are really homophobic and it's not going to change.

Q: Does that bother you?

J: Yes, of course. And I've tried to talk to him and tell him those views are not acceptable, you can't go around saying that.

C: Why not, it's what I feel!

J: You just can't, it's not right to say that about anyone.

C: I don't care, I think its wrong, it should be illegal, and I condemn *battymen*, like Buju Banton [popular reggae artist] preached.

J: What if our son tells us that he is gay when he is older, what would you do then?

C: You know what I would do. I've told you many times before. I'd beat him and tell him 'come out of my house'. Yes, I'd disown him because no son of mine could be that.

J: I would never disown him over that, that's so wrong of you to say that. I would love him and be there for him if he's straight or gay.

C: Well you would have to leave too, I'd put you out of the house with him because I don't want that around me.

J: See what I mean! He's stubborn when it come to that but British men wouldn't be so hostile about gay men because we've grown up with it and just accept it as another part of life. We know it's unacceptable to say those things.

(Clement and Joy, interview location: London, November 2003)

Although Clement and Joy's disagreement was over this issue of sexuality, and the way this could relate to their son in later life, this also reflected wider tensions by newly arrived and established migrants concerning differences in general attitudes to parenting and childrearing decisions. The following extract from our conversation explicates this more fully:

Q: Is there a main source of disagreement in your relationship?

C: Joy is too lenient with the bwoy [boy] and he is going to grow up too soft and sissy. And she doesn't know how to discipline him properly.

J: I do know how to discipline him. I think talking to him and making him understand the reason why I'm telling him off is better than shouting at him like you do.

C: When the bwoy is hard-headed all he needs is two cuffs to the ears and that will make him understand instead of wasting time talking to him. But Joy doesn't want me to discipline him properly. If I even shout at him too rough then she gets upset and says I'm being too hard on him. Where I come from you discipline your children properly, but she doesn't want me to discipline my own child. (ibid.).

Some newly arrived males also believed that a too 'soft' approach to the discipline of boys would encourage their sons to 'turn gay', but – perhaps reflecting a Victorian attitude – they did not have this same concern about their daughters. In some interviews the newly arrived men spoke of the 'confusion' they felt about the 'demanding' and 'contradictory' roles men in Britain were expected to play. They stressed that in the Caribbean men's roles and women's expectations of their men were generally easy to understand, whereas in Britain it was not clear what their female partners wanted or expect from them.

Although most unions between the 'newly arrived' and 'established' were accepted by family and friends, there were also instances of disapproval. Sometimes this was related to perceptions of social class, where the newly arrived was seen as poor and working class. Some newcomers gave examples of 'established' family members expressing hostility and being suspicious of newcomers' intentions. There was the general feeling that these migrants had 'hidden agendas' and were marrying British-born partners in order to gain British citizenship and improve their economic situations. Some relatives appeared generally to expect these unions to be unsuccessful in the long term because of cultural differences, and blamed newcomers for such social problems as the increase of HIV/AIDS across Caribbean communities in England.

Similar issues relating to 'mixing' were evident in some Italian families. Although perhaps not as prominent or problematic as in the Caribbean case, the practice of Italian offspring marrying Italian immigrants was fairly common. The daughters of the early Italian immigrants of the 1930s were often married to men arriving after the Second World War. Often these men found accommodation and work with established Italian families, and this sometimes provided the opportunity for starting intimate relationships. As with the Caribbean examples, these men were sometimes seen to be of lower social status compared with their British-born wives. Of course, there was a degree of truth to this, because they were poorer and urban life was new to them. They were, however, seen as hardworking, which was a valued quality given that often they were joining the wife's family business. Also, given the relatively small size of the Italian community, the fact that they were Italian was seen as good enough and even better when they were from the same villages as the girls' parents. The idea was that continuity with the village of origin would be maintained, and so in general these marriages were not very problematic.

Nonetheless, Giovanna spoke about the differences between her London-based family and her husband's family. She saw her family as being open and cosmopolitan and her husband's family as closed, having been exposed only to village life. She told us that

My husband, his family … my sister is different, she'll come and see us because she grew up here, she knows London, she speaks English. In contrast, his [her husband's] family have been in Trentino and that is it, they've gone as far as Trento to visit the aunt that was there. They haven't been much else in the world and they don't want to, their mentality is what more do you want? And when you're there, when you don't know anything else, it is, what more do you want? You've got your mountains, lovely, but when you have been elsewhere there is a lot more other than Trentino you know?

(Giovanna, interview location: London, March 2004)

As we have also shown in earlier chapters, there have been cases where British-born women of Italian ancestry meet their partners while on holiday in Italy. Many of the young women we interviewed fantasized about going to live in Italy where they thought they could live a life similar to that they experienced on holiday. Above all, they wanted to get away from the control of their immediate families in Britain, and often these relationships became problematic. These British-born women found themselves living in remote parts of Italy where they had few social contacts, and the absence of their own family proved to be a problem because they had no network of support when things with their husbands started to go wrong. They found themselves to be still under familial and community constraints, except that these were not exercised by their own families from whom they had escaped. Like the Caribbean situation, expected and customary gender roles were a cause of tension and division in these unions. The main problem, therefore, that several respondents mentioned was the differences in values they perceived between themselves and their husbands.

Cristina married and then divorced an Italian from Italy. In her interview she made clear the difference she felt existed between British-born Italians and Italians from Italy:

Q: Okay. You married an Italian man the first time. Was it a choice or did it happen by chance … you were looking for an Italian man?
A: No. It happened by chance. … But I wouldn't recommend it for my daughter ever!
Q: To marry an Italian?
A: Never, and live in Italy. To marry an English-born Italian fine, but not to marry an Italian coming from the life she has got here to go and live where I did.
Q: Tell me a bit about that.
A: Two different cultures completely! I went from working for British Airways where I was completely free, to going to live in Italy in a shack with all his parents in the same house. As newly-weds I felt really suppressed. As soon as I had my son, everything changed. No one would babysit. I couldn't get a babysitter and you can't get a stranger to look after your son. I would go out of my door and down the stairs and my mother-in-law would be there. She would say [about baby son] 'He's too hot, he's too cold, and why are you doing this? Why are you doing that?' And I used to answer back at the beginning because

I was English and independent …. I found the Italians friendly but 'backstabbers' and when you're in Italy they always talk about you behind [your back] and I didn't really fit in although I made some very good friends who are still my friends. I hate the culture of men in bars whilst women are at home and that's what he [husband] did. He had his motorbike and Sundays it was on his motorbike. I had my daughter because I knew we were going to split up and I wanted a sister or brother to my son from the same father. Then I just couldn't stand it anymore. We didn't get on and so I came back to England and it was the best thing I could have done for my children.

(Cristina, interview location: London, November 2003)

An activity as simple as the visit 'home' could also be a problem when these couples were from different regions in Italy or from different countries in the Caribbean; there were questions about where to visit, when, for how long, and so forth. The negotiations involved could be fraught with difficulties, as shown in our conversation with Gina:

Q: When you were going on holiday did you go to Puglia or Sicily?
A: That was the problem, I was going to Campania sometimes especially when my mother was still alive but most of the times we went to Puglia to my husband's village. We had a little house there but I didn't like my sister-in-law but we tended to go there more, that was the problem!

(Gina, interview location: Peterborough, March 2004)

Crossing the boundaries within groups that consider themselves as being much the same because they share common identities brings problems, and in transnational contexts families and individuals have to cope as best they can. Sometimes the problem can be over important issues such as how to bring up the children, other times it may be about simple and seemingly inconsequential matters such as having to visit a place to see a disliked sister-in-law. These problems are likely to be more intractable where the mixing is of an inter-ethnic/racial nature.

'Mixed' families across racial and ethnic ties

Individuals in both British-Italian and British-Caribbean communities made such crossings in their intimate relationships, as can be visibly seen on the streets of major British cities and in households up and down the country. The mixing of peoples in the Caribbean from almost every part of the globe since the sixteenth century makes the crossing of racial and ethnic boundaries in Caribbean communities in the region and across the Atlantic seems novel. But, given the waves of invasions and the forward and backward movements of different people in and across the Italian peninsular since the destruction of the Pax Romana, families have been long embedded in the construction of modern Italy. In both sets of communities, therefore, mixing is far from new, and this is also part of their transnational experience in Britain. But, even with such long traditions, these communities' inter-ethnic/racial mixing in Britain has caused tensions and continues to be of concern, much as 'mixed' families do in other communities (see, for example, Callabero *et al.* 2008; Edwards and Callabero 2008).

In this part of our discussion we want to offer some examples from both communities. Emma's recollection is a good starting point, linking the family's past to their present:

> My grandmother favoured my uncle to my dad because my dad is very dark-skinned, jet-black, but my uncle is very light, mixed-raced looks, almost white and I often think that it's bad that my grandmother is like that. The story goes that grandmother sent uncle to one of the top private schools in Jamaica but wouldn't allow my dad to go too because she couldn't afford to send both of them. She sent my uncle because he would have a better chance in life because he was light-skinned. Dad and his mother have never had a close relationship because of that. It has affected us all. My dad and uncle don't get on because of the way their mum treated them and it has affected my relationship with my cousins and we rarely see them [uncle's children] and most of that is to do with the family history. We're the dark side of the family and they're the light side of the family. Maybe things will change with the next generation and there won't be all the isms and schisms that's caused a rift between us.
>
> (Emma, interview location: London, March 2004)

Emma's example is frequently found in Caribbean families with respect to the mixing between black Africans and white Europeans, and well documented in Caribbean studies, literature and folklore. What are not commented upon this side of the Atlantic are the 'mixed' relationships between black Caribbeans, Indo-Caribbeans and South Asians (see, for example, Alibhai-Brown 2001; Datta 2006).

The endogamous tendency in many Indo-Caribbean and South Asian communities prohibits sexual partnerships between individuals from different racial and ethnic communities. Not surprisingly, therefore, our Indo-Caribbean respondents tended to place Caribbeans of African ancestry on the lowest stratum on their hierarchy of racial identities. Sita's story is illustrative of one kind of narrative arising from this situation. She was the daughter of an Afro-Guyanese man and an Indo-Guyanese woman; but Sita's parents had to elope in order to marry, because their respective families were opposed to the relationship. Sita's maternal grandparents felt that her mother was bringing 'shame' on the family by choosing to marry a black man. The increased racial tensions in Guyana between black and Indians during the 1970s made the situation more fraught between Sita's mother and grandmother. Consequently, after her parents married they decided to migrate to Britain, but tension remained between Sita's extended families. On family visits to Guyana Sita's parents travelled separately and they visited their respective family members on separate occasions. Sita was bitter about these families' attitudes and explained that

I don't like to go back [Guyana] because it makes me so unhappy, my parents are unhappy because they have to choose who to stay with and if its my mum's side we visit then dad can't stay and he'll be in a hotel and if its my dad's family, then mum never stayed with them and she'll stay with her family. They never stayed together. We [Sita and her siblings] were caught up in the middle and it's so unfair. Once my mum stayed with dad in the hotel and her family didn't talk to her and said she was disrespectful. It caused too much unhappiness and it was a stressful time. In the end they stopped going.

(Sita, interview location: London, October 2003)

Other respondents in 'mixed' relationships of black Caribbean and South Asian descent also discussed challenges they encountered by family and community members. Marvell, of Caribbean parentage, and Aisha, of Bangladeshi descent, were married and had two primary school age children. Whilst Marvell and Aisha did not themselves view their 'mixed' relationship as a problem or allow their different cultures to affect the ways in which they brought up their children, their marriage created problems for Aisha with her immediate family, extended kin and more generally, within the South Asian community. Aisha said that her family completely disowned her when they found out that she had become engaged and was living with Marvell. After their engagement, Aisha had no further public contact with her family, although she acknowledged that her mother and sister secretly phoned her a couple of times each year. Aisha was afraid to travel to the Southall district in West London in case she met members of her family, kinship group or community, some of whom have threatened to murder her and abduct her children. Aisha noted that in her public life she received 'dirty looks' from people across the diverse South Asian communities and she attributed this to having committed the ultimate taboo of 'marrying black' and having 'mixed' Black/Asian children. In turn, because of these negative experiences that she has encountered from her family and South Asian communities, Aisha decided to reject her family, culture and religion and she took the decision not to teach her children about these matters. Instead, she chose to adopt her husband's ethnic identity and familial cultural practices so that she had a structure of values to pass on to her children.

Similar problems attended mixed relationships between African Caribbeans and West Africans. The problems and tensions between parents and their extended families centred on decisions about the primary culture in which children of these mixed unions should be socialized. The tensions involved may be illustrated from Mayla's experience. A young woman of Nigerian and Jamaican parents, Mayla lived in south-east London. Her grandparents on both sides of her extended families were against her parents' marital union, and Mayla felt that her Nigerian extended family 'look down' on her mother of Jamaican background. She believed that some people in Britain's West African communities viewed Caribbeans as being 'lost' and with 'no culture', resulting from their historical legacy of slavery. Mayla recollected that she herself had been called a 'slave child' by members of her Nigerian family. There was also tension over the question of him passing on his language to his children; Mayla, somewhat regretfully, recollected that

They didn't want to confuse us when we went to nursery. We wouldn't understand. Mum said that it was best because we are living in England, a British society, so trying to teach us two or more languages at that young age would only get us confused and dad didn't challenge this. I think he wanted a peaceful life so he never really tried to teach us ... but I think dad had his own issues, he lost his way and never achieved his parents' expectations to become a top barrister. He disappointed them by marrying a West Indian too. I think he was rebelling against them [parents], it was his way of standing up to them for them being disappointed in his life ... in later years though I know he regrets this ... he never taught us and he so really wanted us to speak his language when we went back [Nigeria]. We recognize a few words but not much.

(Mayla, interview location: London, April 2004)

Mayla's Jamaican kin were equally disappointed by her mother's choice of partner and would have preferred her to marry a Jamaican or a man from another Caribbean country. But as the years passed they appeared to be more accepting of the situation and maintained close contact with Mayla's parents. Perhaps their acceptance could be explained by Mayla's parents' choice to emphasize more the Jamaican cultural heritage in their children's lives, because of the generally open and porous nature of Caribbean culture. Even so, where a Nigerian was involved,

mum's parents weren't pleased at all ... because as far as they were concerned the cultural differences were too big, they didn't understand why she wanted to marry an African when there were plenty of Jamaican men to choose from, and a Nigerian at that, a Ghanaian man would have been just about acceptable, but to fall in love with a Nigerian that's a big no, no .... Mum said right up to the day of the wedding 'your grandmother called and begged me not to do it, she was saying all types of racist things about Nigerians to try and get me to change my mind, ... after the wedding she was like 'Well, you've made your bed ... it will never last, and he'll end up leaving you to marry a Nigerian'. But as time passed, gran has come round and she's admitted that she was wrong. They're still married over 25 years whereas none of her [grandmother's] other children managed to stay married and I think that managed to convince her she was wrong, and it not such a big deal today as it was then.

(Mayla, interview location: London, April 2004)

Mayla acknowledged that it was only on very rare occasions that both the Nigerian and Jamaican sides of her families met socially, and she could recall only one such event – the occasion of her 16th birthday.

'Mixed' marriages between Italian offspring and people from the majority British population or other ethnic groups appear to be more common for men than for women. In close-knit Italian communities such as the Italian community in Bedford, few Italian women marry non-Italian men, whereas the opposite is relatively frequent. Francesca explained that the likelihood of the son having married out is a lot higher. I mean, not marrying an Italian whereas the daughters are brought up exclusively to marry Italian boys. The sons have tended not to, it's very interesting. So the daughter coming back to help her parents is within the construct of having an Italian husband whereas the son being married off or whatever living together with an English girl, it's very different ... 'cos she's English for a start ... their expectations are zero.

Q: So for the parents it would be okay for the sons to marry out?

A: Umm? It's changed. It's become more acceptable. It never was. The pressure was on them to marry Italian girls too but because of the freedom they were allowed, they very often didn't marry Italian women so it's become a lot more acceptable. Interestingly, with English girls, they don't even get married to them because they often live with them nor have children. This is not at all the case with Italian daughters, it's unheard of. They don't live with anybody and they certainly don't have children outside of wedlock whereas the sons do. And it's tolerated.

(Francesca, interview location: London, March 2004)

Although in large cities such as London it was common for Italians to have partners from other ethnic and racial backgrounds, there seemed to be an expectation that the children of offspring would marry Italians. Of course, there were some Italians who did not meet this expectation. Donatella, for example, who married an English-German said that her parents had wanted her to marry an Italian. But they changed their mind after the experience of their other daughter's marriage with a 'real' Italian, meaning an Italian from Italy. Her sister's experience led the parents to the position that

they would not want me to marry an Italian. Not now, now that they know what Italians are really like. When I was little at St Peter's church they tried to palm us off, my primary school days they tried to pair me up with an Italian guy. Then the dream was I would end up with this Italian guy, nothing else mattered just the Italian. It didn't matter who. For a start you weren't meant to go out with boys but if you did then it had to be someone Italian, then they knew I'd never meet a boy so by the time I went to university I met a few guys as you do and then it was really hard introducing them to them, not just 'cos they were English but because they were a boy. I found that whole process really difficult. I didn't want to say 'I'd met this boy, he's English.' So it was really hard, but his mum being German really helped.

(Donatella, interview location: London, November 2003)

For Donatella's parents, the fact that her husband was not totally English helped them to accept him. Her mother thought that the fact that he was half-German made him more European and therefore more similar to Italians. Marrying an English person or another European was considered better than marrying someone from other racial groups, and blacks were seen as totally unacceptable. Donatella's description of her concerns for her parents' feelings on this matter was fairly general; she pointed out that

> at work mum and dad, 'cos they worked in West London, they mixed with lots of Afro-Caribbeans and lots of Asian and Indian groups. But I don't ever think they would have wanted me to go out with a black guy, I think they would have been really upset, I think they would have got over it 'cos their friends were Afro-Caribbean but I don't think they would have coped in the beginning me going out with someone. We have this discussion, I always try to challenge their ideas about this and they say we're not racist, and I hate constructing them as that but they are because of what they're saying is socially unacceptable so yeah.
>
> (Donatella, interview location: London, November 2003)

For non-Italian partners a major problem appeared to be managing the expectations of the Italian partner's family. It was expected that the spouse and the children would spend all their holidays in Italy with family, and the Italian parents expected much more contact than seemed reasonable to non-Italian spouses – and sometimes their Italian partners agreed, as Paulina stressed: 'My partner used to get really angry and say "you see them every two weeks and they still want to see us more" and it was very hard you know to keep both my partner and parents happy' (Paulina, interview location: London, April 2004).

Female Italian respondents married to non-Italian partners expressed surprise at the lack of interference from their in-laws and they also commented on their in-laws' self-sufficiency. This seemed especially the case when they were referring to Italian male family members who had married English women. In a number of interviews with Italian women they critically discussed their English daughters-in-law and sisters-in-law and viewed them in a negative manner. The Italian family members were critical of English female kin members' lack of domestic skills and the little interest they demonstrated in their extended family. Marcella told us that her brother

> married this English girl, Jenny, and she was very immature ... she was in her late twenties when he met her and she was living at home with her parents and I'll never forget when we were visiting once and I remember sitting there when Jenny came home from work and she sat in the kitchen and her mother waited on her. Jenny's meal was in the oven, and she put the meal in front of her and she just sat there eating and when she'd finished it was taken away and then her pudding was put in front of her and I just remembered sitting there looking at this. It was interesting because when they were married, he didn't realize how she had no domestic skills whatsoever and in 25 years of marriage she's never cooked a meal. Luckily my brother, a typical Italian man, he can cook! I don't know why but all the Italian men can cook can't they? He worked quite hard so he didn't have time to do much and she used to go out and just buy stuff from Marks and Spencer's. He just lived on convenience foods you know! It was just

incredible. He'd come home from work quite late about 7pm and he'd have to put the quiche in the microwave. It's just incredible …. When she came over to Italy we used to spend ages cooking like Italians do don't they? When she came to my parent's house she'd lie in bed until 12 noon, I'm not joking! I used to have to take her a cup of tea so she could wake up and come down and my dad was horrified at what she was like and then we all used to talk about her behind her back. She was just lazy, really lazy. God knows why he married her! I just never understood that. I think he kind of respected her because she was a quite serious person but she didn't look after herself, I don't know why.

(Marcella, interview location: London, April 2004)

Some of our Italian respondents explained that their reluctance to marry non-Italians or having family members marrying non-Italians was related to perceived cultural differences. But they were also concerned about the different relationships they felt people of non-Italian origin would experience with their Italian extended family members. This point was borne out in our discussion with Sabrina:

Q: Did you ever think of having an English boyfriend?
A: No, I don't think so. No! Not at all really. Not because they were bad. Mainly I think it was because culture-wise our parents wouldn't be able to accept the person. Even though the English people, their culture isn't so drastic from ours but they wouldn't be able to understand them speak. No, I would never say I would have married an English and, even today to be honest with you, even though everything has changed if my sister-in-law was to marry an English person I'd feel sad.
Q: Really?
A: Yes, I would. Again, not because of anything … I mean I've seen it with my cousin now. She's a lovely girl and she's 32 or something like that and she's met this lovely boy, an English boy. The family had an Italian function which my brother sort of organized and I said 'Where's George?' and she [Wendy] said 'Oh, he doesn't like coming to these things but I'm not going to make excuses for him anymore.' That's what I wouldn't like you know? If I had to have someone he has to be beside me because we are in it together. Like, I presume, if George had a party to go to, my cousin would definitely go and stand beside him and not let him down like that. Do you see what I mean? She's quite sensible really. We say to her 'you marry whoever you like'. But I think she knows that everyone would be more comfortable and so would her partner be more comfortable if it were to be with an Italian man. He would just fit in better. She would fit in better to an Italian family rather than to an English family.

(Sabrina, interview location: Bedford, March 2004)

Two of our interviewees were married to non-Italians and non-English partners who were from different racial or European backgrounds. The first was a person whose grandparents were Italian migrants, and who married a Thai woman, and the second was the case of an Italian woman meeting an Algerian man in London.

They married and went to live in Italy at first and then settled in London due to discrimination against immigrants in Italy. It is worth looking more closely at these two cases.

Dino met his wife while travelling after university; they married in England before her visa was due to expire but the marriage ended in divorce. In the interviews Dino talked little about his failed marriage, but his mother gave her version of the situation. She was concerned about the marriage but she did not oppose it, and she actually organized everything from the restaurant where they had the reception to the dress the bride wore. She attributed the failure of the marriage to cultural differences, particularly the differences about family life. She stressed that the

> family is important to me and to him, but his mother again had a different idea, you know to say go and visit your cousins, she never really showed much interest in wanting to be not part of it, she'd be quite happy if we said come along, but she'd be quite happy to stay on her own, and when somebody can't speak the same language as you it's very difficult to know what they're thinking when they can't express themselves verbally. You can presume it's difficult to know whether she just didn't want to come because she didn't want to, she wanted her independence or to be away from us? I don't know because she would never say, even when there were problems and I knew there were problems … but it is difficult with such a vast difference in culture. We're Europeans and yet I see the difference to the Italian mentality to the English mentality, so you can imagine South East Asian, the climate, the food, everything, just life in general, is so different and really I don't even know 'cos I've never been there. She [the ex-wife] doesn't put an importance on family, I don't know whether it's because her mother died when she was young, I don't know.
>
> (Givoanna, interview location: London, November 2003)

Another example is that of Simona and her Algerian husband. Simona, was born in Italy but lived in London where she worked for an Italian company. Her parents were initially diffident but did not oppose the marriage, and they were open and subsequently quite supportive. The problem for Simona and her husband was that when they became married there were relatively few foreigners in Italy, especially in the small village where they lived. They felt that it was easier for them to live in Britain where they believed they would experience less racism. They had to marry quickly because his visa was running out, but people in her village thought the rush indicated that she was pregnant. Simona was very concerned about the cultural differences between herself and her husband, and this led her to wait for 10 years before having their first child. They were concerned about how to bring up their daughter. Simona felt that, although her husband was not a practising Muslim, he had a strong culture and she also wanted to transmit her own culture to her daughter.

These examples indicate the concern some families expressed about crossing cultural boundaries when forming new families, and sometimes these cultural concerns were as or more important than perceived racial differences. But there is another dimension to the mixing of families in formation.

Opportunities for 'mixed' families

So far we have focused on problems and challenges faced by 'mixed' families, but it is vitally important to acknowledge the opportunities created by these families. After all, mixing along family lines is a great human strength, and is of vital significance in a society as diverse as that of Britain. In the Caribbean situation in Britain, most 'mixed' families were regarded as an unremarkable fact of everyday life and this became an issue mainly when specific problems arose. Indeed, it was quite hard for respondents to focus on our question about opportunities of their mixed families, because of the way they took for granted the 'mixedness' of their families. Sita's narrative illustrates this general point:

Q: How does your Indo- and black Caribbean heritage influence your identity?

A: In my everyday life in England it's not something I think about because there are much more important things to worry about. I don't walk around thinking 'I'm mixed, I'm just plain old Sita from Balham' and mum is mum, dad is dad. But I don't think of us as a mixed-race family but just as a normal family with normal problems like every other families who are black, Indian, white, or Chinese. And don't forget my parents are both from Guyana, and they have that shared history even if mum is Indian and dad is black. It's when other people point it out to me or we have the usual [extended] family drama then I'll remember, 'oh yeh, I'm mixed-race', whatever that means.

(Sita, interview location: London, October 2003)

Additionally, we observed opportunities that resulted from these mixed relationships that were more implicit than explicitly stated. A recurrent theme was that mixed families created greater tolerance of difference amongst family members, as Sita explained:

I'm less judgemental about people compared to my friends and having both [racial] sides of family has helped me think that way because I was raised to see people as people and not to judge people by their skin colour. Anyway, we are all the same under the skin. I have different friends from all walks of life, whereas some of my black friends with Caribbean parents are quite narrow-minded and judgemental and they will keep with their black friends and they will quickly criticize or gossip about someone who doesn't act like them or look like them. My black friends always say 'Sita how you know that person? He's a got …, why are you talking to him?' And I'll say 'I like him, he interests me and he's a laugh'. Besides, I always judge people by their heart, if they have a good heart, then that's good enough for me. I'm interested in doing different things too. They [black friends] will stick to the usual RnB clubs and they're afraid to try anything different. They are much too worried about what others will say if they go against what is expected. But me, I don't care what people think of me and I'll go to gigs, festivals, rock concerts. If I'm curious about it, then I'll go see for myself. I'll try anything once because I just want to try and soak up different ways of lives. I want to experience as much as I can and meet all kinds of people.

(Sita, interview location: London, October 2003)

The offspring of mixed unions appeared to be more able to transmit to their children a better appreciation of cultural differences. For example, Kaya, a young woman of black Caribbean, Indo-Caribbean and white British parentage, was not baptized because her parents believed it was important for her to celebrate the multiple aspects of her racial and ethnic identities. Later as an adult, Kaya could choose which of these identities she wanted to assert as a definition of her identity, but as a child Kaya remembered celebrating both Muslim and Christian religious festivals such as Ramadan and Eid, Christmas and Easter, and practising both faiths.

Richard and Efia, a British-Jamaican and British-Ghanaian couple who lived in London, believed it was important to pass on to their daughter both Jamaican and Ghanaian cultural values and traditions. They appeared to have successfully combined aspects of their respective cultures for their child, including cooking, rituals, and having Jamaican and Ghanaian cultural artefacts in their home and taking holidays in both Ghana and Jamaica. Many 'mixed' families therefore enriched their stocks of cultural and social capital and were able to pass these on to their children. Richard was very aware of their achievement. He told us that

meeting and marrying my wife has been good for me. I didn't know much about Africans or Ghana and their culture and traditions. My eyes and mind are open and I appreciate different cultures and my family to be a part of that. We will raise our children based on both of our Jamaican heritage and Ghanaian heritage. She will get the best of both worlds and her identity will be strongly grounded in the rich cultures of Jamaica and Ghana. Shortly after she was born we had the naming ceremony in the Ghanaian tradition and we felt it was important to do that. Then we have already agreed that my wife's mother will teach her the languages Fante and possibly Ewe as soon as she's old enough to comprehend the language. And I know my mum will want to teach her the Jamaican traditions and she has already weaning her with boiled plantain and ackee so she gets an early taste for Jamaican foods.

(Richard, interview location: London, April 2004)

Grace, another of our interviewees in London, echoed this strong appreciation of dual or multiple or diverse cultural heritage:

[M]um is Jamaican and my dad is Nigerian. I want to acknowledge both sides of my culture and heritage, and I want to acknowledge both sides of my family. I'm lucky because I've spent time with my grandparents and my uncle's family in Nigeria and I see my grandmother and cousins in Jamaica every other year, so I can appreciate both sides of my cultures. Having that experience makes me say 'I'm Nigerian-Jamaican British' or if I'm ticking a box then I usually tick 'Black Other' and write in Nigerian-Jamaican British.

(Grace, interview location: London, January 2004)

Similarly, Sara, an Italian with an Algerian partner, pointed out some of the opportunities created by mixed unions in terms of childrearing and wider family relationships. She stressed that

We have decided to educate our daughter in both our cultures so we try to celebrate Christmas as well as Muslim celebrations. Now she is still young but when she'll grow up perhaps she'll understand what that means. What is positive is that here [in the UK] even at the nursery because they have children from many cultures they speak about all diverse types of cultural celebrations. For example, Chinese celebrations and they have just done the Chinese New Year. They speak about all celebrations and this is positive and this would not have happened if we stayed in Italy.

(Sara, interview location: London, May 2004)

Some women of Italian origin who had married non-Italian partners spoke of the support they gained in their unions with English partners, such as loosening the intense emotional attachments to their parents and being able to pursue their careers and realize their potential. In an earlier chapter we noted how Marcella's elation at shedding her feelings of guilt about her parents was due to her partner's attitude, which gave her confidence. She thought that

Tim really gave me the courage and made me realise how awful my parents were because before then I had just been wracked with guilt non-stop all the time and that was one of the reasons why I couldn't face them and I didn't like seeing them. When he met them he really gave me the courage to understand how dreadful they were! But he never ever said it ... he never said 'Look your Father is this and your Mother is that' ... he never said that. He was just clever I think and he said 'Why do you think you're feeling like that? ... Isn't that a ridiculous thing to do?'

(Marcella, interview location: London, 2004)

As Sara's story illustrated, some couples were aware that a crucial aspect of their strong and positive relationships was the fact that they lived in a tolerant cosmopolitan London. For example, Carla, of Italian background, notes that even though she and her husband had a different upbringing and different religious backgrounds, they felt they had important things in common, because they were both Londoners. She told us that 'although he's not Catholic, he's always been very supportive and has always joined in, so there was never a time when it was as if we had two different religions ... we are both Londoners' (Carla, interview location: London, April 2004).

Moreover, diverse and cosmopolitan London allowed partners in 'mixed' unions to maintain and strengthen transnational links with different parts of the world. Individuals of Italian or Caribbean heritage in Britain whose partners came from Italy or the Caribbean felt that their acts of union reinforced social and cultural links that would otherwise become tenuous over time. Italian and Caribbean partners were generally strongly rooted in transnational networks of family and friends outside Britain and often maintained closer and stronger bonds with immediate kin members who remained behind in Italy and the Caribbean (especially their mother or significant female carers). These factors may also act as a determining factor in the decision to 'return'. In this regard Susanne's reflection on her choice of a partner for life is a fitting statement in bringing this part of our discussion to a close:

> If I hadn't married Everton then probably wouldn't go back so often and I would probably go to Spain for holidays because let's face it, it's cheaper and more convenient than a ten-hour flight! Now I'm married to a fully-fledged Jamaican I have more of a link to the country. It's no longer my parents' history and memory of the place. Now I'm creating my own history in Jamaica with my Jamaican partner and his family who are still out there. Having that link now makes me feel more connected and now I would probably consider returning with him one day and it's not something I would have ever thought about before. I thought my life was pretty much mapped out in Nottingham but now there's another possibility which has opened up and going forward into the future I have more options.
>
> (Susanne, interview location: Nottingham, December 2003)

Conclusion

The overall picture conveyed by accounts of Caribbean and Italian migrants suggests that 'mixed' families present problems of adjustments, but also opportunities to bridge ethnic and racial divides. The opportunities are often taken for granted and rarely considered, and provide a promising area for consideration and research. Unfortunately, it is still the case that it is the problems of 'mixed' families that continue to draw attention, and the social and cultural capital that they create remains relatively neglected. In general, our respondents were more likely to acknowledge and be aware of challenges and constraints faced by 'mixed' family relationships than be cognisant of some of the powerful advantages of 'mixedness'. However, in discussions about the overall aspects and tenor of their everyday lives, it became apparent that these negative factors played a limited role in their families' relationships. Mixed families of any kind appeared to accentuate the positive.

Notes

1 The word 'yard' generally refers to the garden around a Jamaican home, but may also be used to mean 'home' or 'back home', by some migrants and their offspring when describing Jamaica and to a lesser extent other Commonwealth Caribbean countries.
2 Derogatory term used by Caribbeans to refer to homosexual men.

11 Conclusion

Transnational families, policy and research challenges

We have argued that in several important ways members of British families take it for granted that their lives are transnational in terms of their individual interaction within their own immediate families and communities as well as in their contacts with the wider British society. Throughout this book we have suggested that British transnational families formed by post-Second World War migrants and their offspring live with this reality, within a context of 'racial' and ethnic differences. It is part of their everyday experiences. The meeting, mixing, and forming of new families between members from the historic white European populations and relatively new communities also extend aspects of the transnational experience to British society generally, but have not been covered here.

By way of concluding our account of the transnational family dimension or aspects of the post-imperial society that have emerged in Britain, we want to use this final chapter briefly to reflect upon some of the key themes that flow from the accounts offered by our interviewees about their families and their implications for how we may think about future policy and research agendas in relation to transnational family living arrangements and associated factors such as the value of social capital. Three relevant issues order our remarks: the characteristics of the transnational experience within families; the policy implications of these relatively new developments of families across national, racial and ethnic boundaries; and the areas requiring research and further thought.

The transnational experiences of families

In the last six chapters we discussed an array of specific aspects of life that we consider to be of paramount importance in depicting the transnational experiences of families as they were expressed to us by our interviewees. We focused overwhelmingly on families in Britain who have Caribbean and Italian backgrounds. In both cases there are close historical and contemporary links to the British imperial world and the post-imperial Britain that have been emerging over the last half century or so. We have used Britain as the focal point for the meeting of diverse identities, loyalties, belongingness and so forth, because, arguably, Britain is perhaps the most exciting contemporary site where social negotiations are going on as part of the process of reinventing, or reimagining a social order in a post-imperial cast or mould.

We started our empirical analysis of transnational family life with a description of how members have sought to establish themselves and sought to show that they were able to cope with the problems of providing care across distances and national boundaries. Our respondents testified that physical distance did not stop them from carrying out their responsibilities *for* each other and *about* each other. We learnt that these responsibilities were reciprocal, multi-directional, and carried out across generations, irrespective of distance. We also learnt that whilst not exclusively the case, caring tasks are mainly conducted by the female members of families and the kinship group, and that the gender dimension of the transnational family experience warrants particular consideration. The centrality of gender relations within the transnational families that formed part of our research is a recurring theme in most chapters of this book.

Our second area of concern was generational change with respect to migrants, settlement and their offspring. We explored the idea or desire of migrants to 'return' to their homelands as well as the myths that this desire gave rise to in terms of not being fulfilled as well as being reproduced in the consciousness of subsequent generations of offspring. The living space or neighbourhood of settlement came to have significance, and a sense of belongingness developed, linking and rooting families and individuals to particular spaces divided by the boundaries of the nation-state. Friendship networks were seen to be an important part of this process, because these kinds of networks reinforced ethnic and 'racial' bonding even as offspring developed close links with members of the wider British society.

Third, this complex set of negotiations between ethnic and racial, generation and gender, as well as nationality are acted out in a variety of social arenas or social situations. The necessary fluidity that results from the encounters involved were illustrated with respect to sport – a social field of human interaction that has always been meant to minimize social, cultural, ethnic and national distances. In these processes, identities become rather blurred, particularly at the boundaries, and there may therefore be a case to begin to question (in the case of Britain) Barth's (1969) suggestion that it is at the boundaries between ethnic groups that we should look in order to define differences. In other words, we may want to ask whether the boundaries between groups in Britain are not precisely the sites where a degree of what Cohen (1994) called 'fuzziness', or ambiguity, are occurring. Boundary points are further complicated, as we saw in Chapter 8 when we discussed matters of belongingness and the desire to return to 'home' or homeland on the part of both migrants and their offspring, and some instances bringing along partners from other communities in their dreams or their realization of these dreams. Chapter 10 takes up another aspect of this process – namely, families who are composed of members from different 'racial' and ethnic groups and their offspring. These are themes that require further research and consideration.

Families are sometimes portrayed as a panacea for personal and social ills, and our respondents have certainly generally sought to convey to us this powerful aspect of family life. However, as we know, families – whether near or far away – are also a major source for *angst*, pain, and what C. Wright Mills famously called 'personal troubles' (Mills 1970). In Chapter 9, we explored this less than smooth and more troublesome aspect of transnational families. We found an interesting contrast between our two major samples, Caribbeans and Italians, but our findings were not surprising: Italians, like South Asians, uphold close-knit families and extend this across the boundaries of the nation-state; Caribbeans, on the other hand, exhibit a much looser, porous set of relationships, and these too are spread across nation-state boundaries. In either case, however, individuals may find that they need to escape from the iron grip established by the bonds of love and care of the family, and the escape that emigration often provides is not always achieved. The net of love and affection can be cast wide, and is not necessarily a respecter of national boundaries or of distance. In other words, as Castells (2000) suggests, global society carries forward not just the desirable aspects of our lives but also what we may regard as negative aspects.

Some policy implications

It follows, therefore, that the areas of the transnational experiences of families in Britain that we explored in this book have policy implications. This is not just because we were funded by the Economic and Social Research Council (ESRC), which expected us to at least indicate the relevance of our work for identifiable groups. Perhaps of greater significance is the responsibility of which Myrdal (1944, 1970) reminded social analysts and researchers, namely, that good social research must have relevance to contemporary problems, as we noted in Part I of this work. The detailed empirical and theoretical analyses of the responses of our interviewees in Part II of the book demonstrate how relevant patterns of transnational life are to individual members of families, kinship and friendship groups, as well as communities, and indeed nation-states communities. In other words, like all social action, the activity of research is also located within a broadly based moral order in which responsibility is deeply embedded. The question we ask at this point, therefore, is what may be some of the policy implications of our research and the report and analysis given in this book. We want to highlight four of these, and while, like nearly all researchers in the social sciences, we know that they will be ignored, we feel that it is important nonetheless to itemize them here as part of the overall discussion.

First, there is the need for care across state boundaries. Most obvious of these boundaries are those erected by nation-states in a world in which the most significant global boundary is membership of (and exclusion from) the national community. It is within the boundaries of the nation-state that individuals and families are endowed with citizenship rights, and these rebound on, or have implications for, the capacity of family members across boundaries to provide practical care for each other. In the past family members may have cared *about* each other but could do very little beyond remitting funds to needy members 'back home', and assuring them – through letters and photographs – that life in the 'new' country was good.

Today, however, the rapidity of communication, transport, availability of resources and so forth make it possible and practical for such familial responsibilities to be carried out on a scale that was hitherto impossible. Moreover, the wider provision of care in this context can be multi-directional: non-migrants from 'back home' may be able to provide practical assistance and funds to those who migrated and their offspring, as well as receive; there may also be third countries involved in this mutual exchange.

For such undertakings, there is a massive role for the state in the 'homeland' as well as in the country of 'settlement'. In order to achieve 'social welfare citizenship' of the kind envisaged by T. H. Marshall over half a century ago, there may be a need for state-to-state relations to go beyond, or creatively build upon, the United Nations framework.

Second, not only does the organization of such provisions transcend the nation-state construct; it also has implications for identities about our ethnicities, genders and generations. This assertion suggests that we are likely to continue to have questions raised about monoculturalism and multiculturalism for sometime to come. In the first place, the singularity of belongingness required by nationalist ideology (the congruity of folk/people and state/political authority) may have to be yet again delayed or abandoned, and multiple identities, shared identities, long-distance identities accepted as normal for at least a period of time.

Third, given the rising costs of social research, there is a need for the state and its agencies promoting research to find ways of promoting collaborative research beyond state or political blocs. For example, while research within and between scholars and researchers within Europe Union member states is today a priority, given the population composition of the UK, there may be a need to return to something akin to the model that existed during the de-colonization decades of the 1950s and 1960s, when research institutes across the Commonwealth and English-speaking world enjoyed a degree of close individual and institutional collaboration. This would not compromise British scholarship's collaboration with its European partners, but could rather strengthen this, particularly with such partners as France, the Netherlands and Belgium.

Towards a post-national research agenda

These remarks lead to a closer consideration of what might be elements of a possible research agenda around the problematic of transnational families, social capital and associated issues that are at the centre of debates about British society today. We want to highlight just four of these here, and they are not treated in any order of priority; they are all important.

First, our research and analysis have focused on the lives of relatively new minority groups, and while members of the historic majority population featured in our respondents' narratives they were not the focus of the research. But a more all-encompassing net cast to include all British families would involve families from the majority white European communities, as well as families within minority communities who settled in Britain over the last few centuries, such as Jews, East Europeans, the Irish, Africans and others. In particular, the dearth of research into families of African and Asian-Caribbean families (as distinct from African-Caribbean) backgrounds, calls for investigation. In order to appreciate the process or processes of transnational family formation and experiences, it was not necessary to construct such a comprehensive project. However, as the formation and practice of such families are played out in Britain, it may become necessary to have alternative narratives of the kinds of transnational families we describe from the testimonies of members of such collectivities.

Second, we have not attempted to explore the crucial questions of how transnational families impact on the economic and political dimensions of the transnational experience. This is partly because there is already considerable research on these dimensions, with respect to nationalism, intellectual cross-currents, investments and transnational networks (Fuglerund 1999; Levitt 2001; Robins and Aksoy 2001; Ostergaard-Nielsen 2003). Nonetheless, there is a need to link these discussions, and in particular to show how transnational families facilitate political participation and economic processes (Martiniello and Lafleur 2008; Portes *et al.* 2008). Such a contribution would be at the discrete, micro-level, of social analysis, and may be considered to be the province of biography and autobiography. We suggest that these veins of the overall process will enrich any future programme on British transnational families.

A third matter that will need to be taken on board in any research agenda for the future is that of longevity. In other words, while we live in interesting times and are seeing and experiencing the fluidity and autonomy of families across boundaries of every kind – national, racial, ethnic, preferences/choice, generation and so forth – we may want to ask how long this is likely to last. The 'open society' that is post-imperial Britain may not endure. Tolerance, acceptance, embracing 'the other' could give way to their opposites in a cruel Hegelian dialectical logic, and take us back to a world of hard and fixed boundaries. We need, therefore to explore more critically the conditions necessary for the thriving of a society in which a 'thousand flowers bloom' together. In this regard, the formation of intimate relationships – friendship networks, families across the boundaries along any exclusive lines – constitutes key areas for future investigations.

The core themes of this book resonate with ongoing debates in a wide range of societies about the role of transnational processes in shaping the everyday experiences of significant numbers of people across the globe. In presenting the main findings of our research we have sought both to contribute to these debates and to suggest how the kind of grounded research that we have undertaken in relation to transnational families can help us to understand these processes in a more systematic manner. It is through old and imaginative research on these and related issues that we can help to inform public debate about a phenomenon that is likely to shape a wide range of societies for the future.

Bibliography

Abenaty, F. (2000) 'St Lucians and Migration: Migrant Returnees, Their Families and St Lucian Society', unpublished PhD Thesis, London: South Bank University.

Abenaty, F. (2001) 'The Dynamics of Return Migration to St. Lucia', in H. Goulbourne and M. Chamberlain (eds), *Caribbean Families in Britain and the Trans-Atlantic World*, London: Macmillan, 170–87.

Ackers, H. L. and Stalford, H. E. (2004) *A Community for Children? Children, Citizenship and Internal Migration in the EU*, Aldershot: Ashgate.

Aleinikoff, A. (2002) *Citizenship Policies for an Age of Migration*, Washington, DC: Carnegie Endowment for International Peace.

Alibhai-Brown, Y. (2001) *Mixed Feelings: The Complex Lives of Mixed Race Britons*, London: Women's Press.

Allan, G. and Adams, R. (eds) (1999) *Placing Friendships in Context*, Cambridge: Cambridge University Press.

Ahmed, W. I. U. (ed) (1993) *'Race' and health in contemporary Britain*, Buckingham: Open University Press.

Ahmed, W. I. U. and Atkin, K. (eds) (1996) *'Race' and community care*, Buckingham: Open University Press.

Anderson, B. (2006) *Imagined Communities: Reflections on the Origin and Spread of Nationalism*, new edn, London: Verso.

Ansell, A. E. (1997) *New Right, New Racism: Race and Reaction in the United States and Britain*, New York: New York University Press.

Anthias, F. (2007) 'Ethnic Ties: Social Capital and the Question of Mobilisability', *Sociological Review*, 55, 4: 788–805.

Anthias, F. and Yuval-Davies, N. (1992) *Racialised Boundaries: Race, Nation, Gender, Colour, and Class and the Anti-Racists Struggle*, London: Routledge.

Anwar, M. (1979) *The myth of return*, London: Heinemann.

Arneil, B (2006) *Diverse Communities: The Problem with Social Capital*, Cambridge: Cambridge University Press.

Back, L. and Solomos, J. (eds) (2000) *Theories of Race and Racism: A Reader*, London and New York: Routledge.

Baldassar, L. (2001) *Visits Home: Migration Experiences Between Italy and Australia*, Melbourne: Melbourne University Press.

Banton, M. (1967) *Race Relations*, London: Tavistock.

Banton, M. (2006) 'Perspectives on race relations research', Talk given at the Keyworth Centre, London South Bank University (March).

Baron, S., Field, J. and Schuller, T. (eds) (2000) *Social Capital: Critical Perspectives*, Oxford: Oxford University Press.

Barrow, C. (1996) *Family in the Caribbean: Themes and Perspectives*, London: James Currey.

Barrow, J. (1982) 'West Indian Families: An Insider's Perspective', in R. N. Rapoport, M. P. Fogerty and R. Rapoport (eds), *Families in Britain*, London: Routledge, 220–32.

Barth, F. (ed.) (1969) *Ethnic Groups and Boundaries*, London: George Allen and Unwin.

Bashi, V. (2007) *Survival of the Knitted: Immigrant Social Networks in a Stratified World*, Stanford: Stanford University Press.

Bauböck, R. (2003) 'Towards a Political Theory of Transnationalism', *International Migration Review*, 37, 3: 700–23.

Bauböck, R. (ed.) (2006) *Migration and Citizenship: Legal Status, Rights and Political Participation*, Amsterdam: Amsterdam University Press.

Bauer, E. and Thompson, P. (2006) *Jamaican Hands across the Atlantic*, Kingston: Ian Randle Publishers.

Bauman, G. (1996) *Contesting Cultures: Discourses of Identity in Multi-Cultural London*, Cambridge: Cambridge University Press.

Beck, U. (1992) *Risk Society: Towards a New Modernity*, London: Sage.

Beck, U. and Beck-Gernsheim, E. (2002) *Individualization*, London: Sage.

Beck-Gernsheim, E. (2007) 'Transnational Lives, Transnational Marriages: A Review of the Evidence from Migrant Communities in Europe', *Global Networks*, 7, 3: 271–88.

Benhabib, S. (2002) *The Claims of Culture: Equality and Diversity in the Global Era*, Princeton: Princeton University Press.

Bentley, A. (1908) *The Process of Government*, Cambridge, MA: Harvard University Press.

Benyon, J. and Solomos, J. (eds) (1987) *The Roots of Urban Unrest*, Oxford: Pergamon Press.

Benyon, J. and Solomos, J. (1988) 'The Simmering Cities: Urban Unrest During the Thatcher Years', *Parliamentary Affairs*, 41, 3: 402–22.

Berrington, A. (1994) 'Marriage and Family Formation among the White and Ethnic Minority Populations in Britain', *Ethnic and Racial Studies*, 17, 3: 517–46.

Berrington, A. (1996) 'Marriage patterns and inter-ethnic unions', in D Coleman and J Salt (eds), *Ethnicity in the 1991 Census: demographic characteristics of the ethnic minority population*, vol 1, London: OPCS.

Bianchi, S. M. and Robinson, J. (1997) '"What did you do today?" Children's use of time, family composition and acquisition of cultural capital', *Journal of Marriage and the Family*, 59: 332–44.

Birch, A. H. (1993) *The concepts and theories of modern democracy*, London: Routledge.

Bleich, E. (2003) *Race Relations in Britain and France: Ideas and Policymaking Since the 1960s*, Cambridge: Cambridge University Press.

Bloch, A. (2002) *The Migration and Settlement of Refugees in Britain*, Basingstoke: Palgrave Macmillan.

Bloemraad, I. (2007) 'Unity in Diversity?', *Du Bois Review: Social Science Research on Race*, 4, 2: 317–36.

Bloemraad, I., Korteweg, A. and Yurdakul, G. (2008) 'Citizenship and Immigration: Multiculturalism, Assimilation, and Challenges to the Nation-State', *Annual Review of Sociology*, 34, 1: 153–79.

Bornat, J., Dimmock, B., Jones, D. and Peace, S. (1999) 'Generational Ties in the 'New' Family: Changing Contexts for Traditional Obligations', in E. B. Silva and C. Smart (eds), *The 'New' Family*, London: Sage, 248–62.

Boswell, C. (2007) 'Theorising Migration Policy: Is There a Third Way?', *International Migration Review*, 41, 1: 75–100.

Bottignolo, B. (1985) *Without a Bell Tower. A Study of the Italian Immigrants in South-West England*, Rome: Centro Studi Emigrazione.

Bourdieu, P. (1997) 'The forms of capital', in J. G. Richardson (ed), *Handbook of theory and research for the sociology of education*, Slough: Greenwood Press, 241–58.

Bourdieu, P and Passeron, J-C. (1990) *Reproduction in Education, Society and Culture*, London: Sage.

Brah, A. (1996) *Cartographies of Diaspora: Contesting Identities*, London: Routledge.

Brodber, E. (1974) *The Abandonment of Children in Jamaica*, Institute of Social and Economic Research, Kingston: University of West Indies Press.

Brown, C. (1984) *Black and white Britain*, London: Policy Studies Institute.

Bryceson, D. and Vuorela, U. (eds) (2002) The Transnational Family: New European Frontiers and Global Networks, Oxford: Berg.

Buijs, G. (ed.) (1993) *Migrant Women: crossing boundaries and changing identities*, Oxford: Berg.

Burman, J. (2002) 'Remittance; Or, Diasporic Economies of Yearning', *Small Axe*, 12, 2: 49–71.

Caballero, C., Edwards, R. and Puthussery, S. (2008) *Parenting 'Mixed' Children: Negotiating Differences and Belonging in Mixed Race, Ethnicity and Faith Families*, York: Joseph Rowntree Foundation.

Caballero, C., Edwards, R. and Smith, D. (2008) 'Cultures of Mixing: Understanding Partnerships across Ethnicity', *21st Century Society*, 39, 1: 49–63.

Cabinet Office (2000) *Social Capital: A Discussion Paper*, London: Performance and Innovation Unit.

Calhoun, C. J., Price, R. and Timmer, A. (eds) (2002) *Understanding September 11*, New York: New Press.

Callender, C. (1997) *Education for Empowerment: The Practice and Philosophies of Black Teachers*, London: Trentham Books.

Campbell, C. and McLean, C. (2002) Ethnic Identity, Social Capital and Health Inequalities: Factors Shaping African-Caribbean Participation in Local Community Networks', Elsevier Science. Available at: http://eprints.lse.ac.uk/181/1/ethnic_identities.pdf (accessed 30 September, 2007).

Cantle, T. (2001) *Community Cohesion: A Report of the Independent Review*, London: Home Office.

Carling, J. (2002) 'Migration in the Age of Involuntary Immobility: Theoretical Reflections and Cape Verdean Experiences', *Journal of Ethnic and Migration Studies*, 28, 1: 5–42.

Carter, B., Harris, C. and Joshi, S. (1987) 'The 1951–55 Conservative Goverment and the Racialization of Black Immigration', *Immigrants and Minorities*, 6, 3: 335–47.

Castells, M. (2000) *The Rise of the Network Society*, 2nd edn, Oxford: Blackwell.

Castles, S. (2000) *Ethnicity and Globalization: From Migrant Worker to Transnational Citizen*, London: Sage.

Castles, S. (2004) 'The Factors that Make and Unmake Migration Policies', *International Migration Review*, 38, 3: 852–84.

Castles, S. (2007) 'Twenty-First-Century Migration as a Challenge to Sociology', *Journal of Ethnic and Migration Studies*, 33, 3: 351–71.

Castles, S. and Miller, M. J. (2009) *The Age of Migration: International Population Movements in the Modern World*, 4th edn, Basingstoke: Palgrave Macmillan.

Cavallaro, R. (1981) *Storie Senza Storia. Indagine Sull'emigrazione Calabrese in Gran Bretagna*, Rome: Centro Studi Emigrazione.

Chafetz, J. S. (1997) 'Feminist Theory and Sociology: Underutilized Contributions for Mainstream Theory', *Annual Review of Sociology*, 23: 97–120.

Chamberlain, M. (2006) *Narratives of Exile and Return*, New Brunswick: Transaction Publishers.

Charles, N., Aull Davies, C. and Harris, C. (2008) *Families in Transition: Social Change, Family Formation and Kin Relationships*, Bristol: The Policy Press.

Chevannes, B. (1996) 'Swimming against the Tide: The Real Position of Caribbean Pen', Paper presented at the Caribbean Males: An Endangered Species Conference, University of West Indies at Mona, 12–14 April.

Chevannes, B. (2002), *Learning to be a Man: culture, socialization and gender identity in five Caribbean communities*, Kingston: University of West Indies Press.

Chistolini, S. (1986) *Donne Italo-Scozzesi; tradizione e cambiamento*, Rome: Centro Studi Emigrazione.

Christou, A. (2002) 'Greek American Return Migration: Constructions of Identity and Re-constructions of Place', *Migration Studies: International Journal of Migration Studies*, 39, 145: 201–29.

Christou, A. (2006) 'Deciphering Diaspora-Translating Transnationalism: Family Dynamics, Identity Constructions and the Legacy of "Home" in Second-Generation Greek-American Return Migration', *Ethnic and Racial Studies*, 29, 6: 1040–56.

Clarke, E. (1957) *My Mother Who Fathered Me*, London: George Allen and Unwin.

Clement, G. (1996) *Care, Autonomy and Justice: Feminism and the Ethic of Care*, Boulder, CO: Westview Press.

Cohen, J. (1999) 'Trust, Voluntary Association and Workable Democracy: the Contemporary American Discourse on Civil Society', in M. Warren (ed.), *Democracy and Trust*, Cambridge: Cambridge University Press.

Cohen, R. (1994) *Fuzzy Frontiers of Identity: The British Case and the Others*, London: Longman.

Cohen, R. (1996) 'Diasporas and the Nation-State: From Victims to Challengers', *International Affairs*, 72, 3: 507–20.

Cohen, R. (2008) *Global Diasporas: An Introduction*, 2nd edn, London: UCL Press.

Coleman, J. S. (1990) *Foundations of Social Theory*, London: Harvard University Press.

Coleman, J. S. (1988) 'Social capital in the creation of human capital', *American Journal of Sociology*, 94 (supplement), S95-S120.

Colpi, T. (1991) *The Italian Factor: The Italian Community in Great Britain*, London: Mainstream.

Colpi, T. (1993) 'Origins and Campanilismo in Bedford's Italian Community', in L. Sponza and A. Tosi (eds), 'A Century of Italian Emigration to Britain 1880–1980s', Supplement to *The Italianist*, 13, 59–77.

Colucci, M. (2002) 'L'emigrazione italiana in Gran Bretagna nel secondo dopoguerra: il caso di Bedford (1951–60)', *Dimensioni e problemi della ricerca storica*, 1: 235–272.

Commission for Racial Equality (2004) 'Few Black Friends for Whites', *BBC News*. Available at: http:news.bbc.co.uk/1/hi/uk/3906193.stm (accessed 20 March, 2009).

Commission for Racial Equality (2005) *Commission for Integration and Cohesion: A Response by the Commission for Racial Equality*, London: Commission for Racial Equality.

Commission for Racial Equality (2006) *30: At the Turning of the Tide*, London: Commission for Racial Equality.

Conway, D. (1993) 'Rethinking the Consequence of Remittances for Eastern Caribbean Development', *Caribbean Geography*, 4: 116–30.

Cooper, C. (1995) *Noises in the Blood: Orality, Gender and the 'Vulgar' Body of Jamaican Popular Culture*, London: Macmillan.

Cornell, S. and Hartmann, D. (1998) *Ethnicity and Race: Making Identities in a Changing World*, Thousand Oaks, CA: Pine Forge Press.

Cowan, H. and Goulbourne, H. (2001) 'From Academe to Polity: Tensions in Conducting Policy and Community Research', in H. Goulbourne (ed.), *Race and Ethnicity: Critical Concepts in Sociology*, 3, London: Routledge, 400–15.

Dahl, R. (1961) *Who Governs? Democracy and power in an American city*, New Haven and London: Yale University Press.

Daniel, W. (1968) *Racial discrimination in Britain*, Harmondsworth: Penguin.

Datta, T (2006) 'Is This the Last Taboo?', *BBC News*. Available at: http://news.bbc.co.uk/1/hi/magazine/5071026.stm (accessed 12 February, 2009).

Datta, T (2007) 'The Elephant in the Room', Commission for Racial Equality. Available at: http://mixedness.millipedia.net/Default.aspx.LocID-0hgnew0xi.RefLocID-0hg0110hg01l001.Lang-EN.htm (accessed 12 February, 2009).

De Vault, M. L. (1996) 'Talking Back to Sociology: Distinctive Contributions of Feminist Methodology', *Annual Review of Sociology*, 22, 1: 29–50.

Dench, G. (1986) *Minorities in the Open Society: Prisoners of Ambivalence*, London: Routledge and Kegan Paul.

Denham, J. (2001) *Building Cohesive Communities: A Report of the Ministerial Group on Public Order and Community Cohesion*, London: Home Office.

Di Leonardo, M. (1992) 'The Female World of Cards and Holidays: women, families and the work of kinship', in B. Thorne and M. Yalom (eds), *Rethinking the Family: some feminist questions*, Boston: Northern University Press.

Dias-Briquets, S. and Weintraub, S. (eds) (1991) *Migration, Remittances and Small Business Development: Mexico and Caribbean Basin Countries*, Boulder, CO: Westview Press.

Driessen, G. (2001) 'Ethnicity, forms of capital and educational achievement', *International Review of Education*, 47, 6: 513–38.

Du Bois, W. E. B. (1903) *The Souls of Black Folk: Essays and Sketches*, London: Longmans, Green.

Du Bois, W. E. B. (1973) *The Philadelphia Negro: a social study*, first published 1899, with a new Introduction by H. Aptheker, Millwood, New York: Kraus-Thompson.

Edwards, J., Oakley, A. and Popya, J. (1999) 'Service Users and Providers' Perspectives on Welfare Needs', in F. Williams (ed.), *Welfare Research: a critical review*, London: UCL Press.

Edwards, R. (2004) 'Present and Absent in Troubling Ways: Families and Social Capital Debates', *Sociological Review*, 52, 1: 1–21.

Edwards, R. and Caballero, C. (2008) 'What's In A Name? An Exploration of the Significance of Personal Naming of "Mixed" Children for Parents from Different Racial, Ethnic and Faith Backgrounds', *Sociological Review*, 56, 1: 39–59.

Edwards, R. and Gillies, V. (2005) 'Resources in Parenting: Access to Capitals Project Report', Families & Social Capital ESRC Research Group Working Paper No. 14, London: South Bank University.

Edwards, R., Franklin, J. and Holland, J. (2003) 'Families and Social Capital: Exploring the Issues', Families & Social Capital ESRC Research Group Working Paper No. 1, London: South Bank University.

Ehrenreich, B. and Hochschild, A. (eds) (2003) *Global Woman: Nannies, Maids and Sex Workers in the New Economy*, London: Granta Books.

Faist, T. (2000) 'Transnationalization in International Migration: Implications for the Study of Citizenship and Culture', *Ethnic and Racial Studies*, 23, 2: 189–222.

Fanon, F. (1968) *Black Skins, White Masks*, London: Macgibbon & Kee.

Fanon, F. (1970) *A Dying Colonialism*, London: Penguin.

Faulkner, D. (2004) *Civil Renewal, Diversity and Social Capital in Multi-Ethnic Britain*, London: Runnymede Trust.

Favell, A. (2001) *Philosophies of Integration: Integration and the Idea of Citizenship in France and Britain*, 2nd edn, Basingstoke: Palgrave.

Fevre, R. (2004) *Social Capital and the Participation of Marginalised Groups in Government*, ESRC Funded Project, R000249410, Swindon: ESRC.

Field, J. (2003) *Social Capital*, London: Routledge.

Finch, J. (1989a) *Family Obligation and Social Change*, Cambridge: Polity Press.

Finch, J. (1989b) 'Kinship and friendship', in R. Jowell, S. Witherspoon and L. Brook (eds) *British Social Attitudes. Special International Report*, Aldershot: Gower.

Finch, J. and Groves, D. (eds) (1983) *A Labour of Love: Women, Work, and Caring*, London: Routledge.

Finch, J. and Mason, J. (1993) *Negotiating Family Responsibilities*, London: Routledge.

Fisher, B. and Tronto, J. (1990) 'Towards a Feminist Theory of Caring', in E. K. Abel and M. K. Nelson (eds), *Circles of Care: work and identity in women's lives*, New York: New York Press.

Fog Olwig, K. (1993) 'The Migrant Experience: Nevisian women at home and abroad', in J. Momsen (ed), *Women and change in the Caribbean*, London: James Curry.

Foner, N. (1979) *Jamaica Farewell: Jamaican Migrants in London*, London: Routledge and Kegan Paul.

Foner, N. (ed.) (2001) *Islands in the City: West Indian Migration to New York*, Berkeley: University of California Press.

Foner, N. (2002) 'Second-Generation Transnationalism, Then and Now', in P. Levitt and M. Waters (eds), *The Changing Face of Home: the transnational lives of the second generation*, New York: Russell Sage Foundation.

Foner, N. (ed.) (2005) *Wounded City: The Social Impact of 9/11*, New York: Russell Sage Foundation.

Fordham, S and Ogbu, J (1986) 'Black Student Success: Coping with the Burden of "Acting White"', *Urban Review*, 18, 1: 176–206.

Fortier, A. M. (2000) *Migrant Belongings: Memory, Space, Identity*, Oxford: Berg.

Fouron, G. and Schiller, N. G. (2001) 'All in the Family: Gender, Transnational Migration and the Nation-State', *Identities*, 7, 4: 539–82.

Fraser, S. (ed.) (1995) *The Bell Curve Wars: Race, Intelligence and the Future of America*, New York: Basic Books.

Fuglerund, O. (1999) *Life on the Outside: The Tamil Diaspora and Long Distance Nationalism*, London: Pluto Press.

Furstenberg, F. (2005) 'Neighbours and Social Capital', unpublished keynote address at International Conference, Wither Social Capital?, ESRC Research Group, London: South Bank University.

Gabaccia, D. and Iacovetta, F. (eds) (2002) *Women, Gender, and Transnational lives: Italian workers of the world*, Toronto: Toronto University Press.

Ganga, D. (2006) 'From Potential Returnees into Settlers: Nottingham's Older Italians', *Journal of Ethnic and Migration Studies*, 32, 8: 1395–413.

Gann, N. (1998) 'Improving school governance', London: Falmer Press.

Gardner, K. (2002) *Age, Narrative and Migration: The Life Course and Life Histories of Bengali Elders in London*, Oxford: Berg.

Gardner, K. (2006) 'The Transnational Work of Kinship and Caring: Bengali-British Marriages in Historical Perspective', *Global Networks*, 6, 4: 373–87.

Gardner, K. and Grillo, R. (2002) 'Transnational households and rituals: an overview', *Global Networks: a journal of transnational affairs*, July, 2, 3: 179–90.

Giddens, A. (1992) *Modernity and Self-identity: self and society in the late modern age*, Cambridge: Polity Press.

Giddens, A. (2003) *Runaway World: how globalisation is reshaping our lives*, 2nd ed. London: Routledge.

Ginsborg, P. (2003) *Italy and its Discontents 1980–2001*, London: Penguin Books.

Glick-Schiller, N. (1997) 'The Situation of Transnational Studies', *Identities*, 4, 2: 155–66.

Glick-Schiller, N. (2004) 'Transnationality', in D. Nugent and J. Vincent (eds), *A Companion to the Anthropology of Politics*, Malden: Blackwell.

Glick-Schiller, N., Basch, L., Szanton-Blanc, C. (1992) *Towards a Transnational Perspective on Migration*, New York: New York Academy of Sciences.

Gmelch, G. (1980) 'Return Migration', *Annual Review of Anthropology*, 9: 135–59.

Goring, B. (2004) 'Perspectives of UK Caribbean Parents on Schooling and Education: Change and Continuity', unpublished PhD Thesis, London: South Bank University.

Goulbourne, H. (1990) 'The Contribution of West Indian Groups to British Politics', in H. Goulbourne (ed.), *Black Politics in Britain*, London: Avebury, 95–114.

Goulbourne, H. (1991) *Ethnicity and Nationalism in Post-Imperial Britain*, Cambridge: Cambridge University Press.

Goulbourne, H. (1998) *Race Relations in Britain Since 1945*, Basingstoke: Palgrave Macmillan.

Goulbourne, H. (1999) 'The transnational character of Caribbean kinship in Britain', in S. McRae (ed), *Changing Britain: families and households in the 1990s*, Oxford: Oxford University Press.

Goulbourne, H. (2001), 'General Introduction', in H. Goulbourne (ed.), *Race and Ethnicity: Critical Concepts in Sociology*, 4 vols, London: Routledge, 1–13.

Goulbourne, H. (2002) *Caribbean Transnational Experience*, London: Pluto Press.

Goulbourne, H. (2006) 'A Distrust of Politics?: People of African Heritage in Britain and the Atlantic World', in W. Berthomiere and C. Chivallon (eds), *Les Diasporas dans le monde contemporain*, Paris: Karthala, 377–90.

Goulbourne, H. (2008a) 'Families in Black and Minority Ethnic Communities and Social Capital: past and continuing false prophesies in social studies', in R. Edwards (ed.) *Researching Families and Communities: social and generational change*, London: Routledge, ch. 5.

Goulbourne, H. (2008b) 'Race, ethnicity and development in the Atlantic world', in A. Bonnett and C. Holder (eds) *Continuing perspectives on the Black Diaspora*, Lanham: University of America Press, ch 2.

Goulbourne, H. and Chamberlain, M. (eds) (2001) *Caribbean Families in Britain and the Trans-Atlantic World*, Basingstoke: Macmillan Caribbean.

Goulbourne, H., Cowen, H. and Owen, D. (1995) *The Needs of the African Caribbean Community in Coventry: a report*, Cheltenham: University of Gloucestershire.

Goulbourne, H. and Solomos, J. (2003) 'Families, Ethnicity and Social Capital', *Social Policy and Society*, 2, 4, 329–38.

Gray, A. (2005) 'The Changing Availability of Grandparents as Carers and its Implications for Childcare Policy in the UK', *Journal of Social Policy*, 34, 4: 557–77.

Griffiths, M. (1995) *Feminism and the Self: The Web of Identity*, London: Routledge.

Grillo, R. (2007) 'Betwixt and between: Trajectories and Projects of Transmigration', *Journal of Ethnic and Migration Studies*, 33, 2: 199–217.

Grillo, R. (ed.) (2008) *The Family in Question: Immigrant and Ethnic Minorities in Multicultural Europe*, Amsterdam: Amsterdam University Press.

Guiraudon, V. and Lahav, G. (eds) (2007) *Immigration Policy in Europe: The Politics of Control*, London: Routledge.

Hall, S., Critcher, T., Jefferson, T., Clarke, J. and Roberts, B. (1978) *Policing the Crisis: Mugging, the State and Law and Order*, Basingstoke: Macmillan.

Halpern, D. (2005) *Social Capital*, London: Polity Press.

Haritaworn, J. (2009) 'Hybrid Border-Crossers? Towards a Radical Socialisation of "Mixed Race"', *Journal of Ethnic and Migration Studies*, 35, 1: 115–32

Harker, J. (2007) 'Role Models Should Come from the Home, not the TV', *Guardian*, 14 August.

Harpalani, V. (2001) 'Identity and School Adjustment: Questioning the "Acting White" Assumption', *Educational Psychologist*, 36, 1: 21–30.

Harpalani, V. (2004) *Genetic, Racial and Cultural Determinism in Discourses on Black Athletes*, unpublished paper presented at the American Sociological Association, 14 August, San Francisco. Available at: http://www.allacademic.com/meta/p110091_index. html(accessed 18 February, 2009).

Harris, C. (1988) 'Images of Blacks in Britain: 1930–60', in S. Allen. and M. Macey (eds), *Race and Social Policy*, London: Economic and Social Research Council.

Hart, V. (1978) *Distrust and Democracy: Political Distrust in Britain and America*, London: Cambridge University Press.

Hemmings, C. (2005) 'Telling Feminist Stories', *Feminist Theory*, 6, 2: 115–39.

Herrnstein, R. J. and Murray, C. (1994) *The Bell Curve: Intelligence and Class Structure in American Life*, New York: Free Press.

Holland, J., Reynolds, T. and Weller, S. (2007) 'Transitions, Networks and Communities: The Significance of Social Capital in the Lives of Children and Young People', *Journal of Youth Studies*, 10, 1: 101–20.

Holmes, C. (1988) *John Bull's Island*, Basingstoke: Macmillan.

Home Office (2005) *Improving Opportunity, Strengthening Society: The Government's Strategy to Increase Race Equality and Community Cohesion*, London: Home Office.

Hussain, A. M. (2001) *British Immigration Policy Under the Conservative Government*, Aldershot: Ashgate.

Irwin, S. (1999) 'Resourcing the Family: gendered claims and obligations and issues of explanation', in E. B Silva and C. Smart (eds), *The 'New' Family*, London: Sage.

Jacob, J. D. (1986) *Black Politics and Urban Crisis in Britain*, Cambridge: Cambridge University Press.

Jacoby, R. and Glaubermann, N. (eds) (1995) *The Bell Curve Debate: History, Documents, Opinions*, New York: Times Books.

James, C. and Harris, W. (1993) *Inside Babylon: The Caribbean Diaspora in Britain*, London: Verso.

Kasinitz, P., Mollenkopf, J. H., Waters, M. C. and Holdaway, J. (2008) *Inheriting the City: The Children of Immigrants Come of Age*, Cambridge, MA: Harvard University Press.

King, R. (1977) 'Bedford: the Italian connection', *Geographical Magazine*, 49, 7: 442–9.

King, R. (1979) 'Return Migration: A Review of Some Case-Studies from Southern Europe', *Mediterranean Studies*, 1, 2: 3–30.

King, R. (ed.) (1986) *Return Migration and Regional Economic Problems*, London: Croom Helm.

King, R. (2000) 'Generalisation from the History of Return Migration', in B. Ghosh (ed.), *Return Migration: Journey of Hope or Despair?*, Geneva: IOM and UN.

King. R. and Christou, A. (2008) 'Cultural Geographies of Counter-Diasporic Migration Diaspora', SCMR Working Paper Series, University of Sussex.

King, R. and King, P. D. (1977) 'The spatial evolution of the Italian community in Bedford', *East Midland Geographer*, 6, 7: 337–45.

Komter, A. E. (2005) *Social solidarity and the gift*, Cambridge: Cambridge University Press.

Kushner, T. (2009) *Anglo-Jewry since 1066: Place, Locality and Memory*, Manchester: Manchester University Press.

Laslett, B. (2007) 'Feminist Sociology in the Twentieth-Century United States: Life Stories in Historical Context', in C. Calhoun. (ed.), *Sociology in America: A History*, Chicago: University of Chicago Press, 480–502.

Lassman, P. and Velody, I. (eds) (1988) *Max Weber's 'Science as a Vocation'*, London: Unwin Hyman.

Levitt, P. (1998) 'Social Remittances: Migration Driven Local-Level Forms of Cultural Diffusion', *International Migration Review*, 32, 4: 926–48

Levitt, P. (2001) *The Transnational Villagers*, Berkeley: University of California Press.

Levitt, P. and Waters, M. (eds) (2002) *The Changing Face of Home: The Transnational Lives of the Second Generation*, New York: Russell Sage Foundation.

Levitt, P. and de la Delera, R. (2003) 'Transnational Migration and the Redefinition of the State: Variations and Explanations' *Ethnic and Racial Studies*, 26, 4: 587–611.

Levitt, P. and Schiller, N. G. (2004) 'Conceptualizing Simultaneity: A Transnational Social Field Perspective on Society', *International Migration Review*, 38, 3: 1002–39.

Levitt, P. and Jaworsky, B. N. (2007) 'Transnational Migration Studies: Past Developments and Future Trends', *Annual Review of Sociology*, 33, 1: 129–56.

Lewis, L. L. (1993) *W. E. B. Du Bois: Biography of a Race, 1868–1919*, New York: Henry Holt and Company.

Lummis, T. (1987) *Listening to History: the authenticity of oral evidence*, London: Hutchinson.

McGhee, D. (2008) *The End of Multiculturalism? Terrorism, Integration and Human Rights*, Maidenhead: Open University Press.

Mackenzie, C. and Stoljar, N. (eds) (2000) *Relational Autonomy: Feminist Perspectives on Autonomy, Agency and the Social Self*, New York: Oxford University Press.

Macpherson, W. (1999) *The Stephen Lawrence Inquiry*, London: HMSO.

McRae, S. (1997) (ed.) *Changing Britain: Families and Households in the 1990s*, Oxford: Oxford University Press.

Maffioletti, M. (2004) Director, Centro Studi Emigrazione Roma, interview with E. Zontini, 15 January.

Malik, K. (1996) *The Meaning of Race*, London: Macmillan.

Malinowski, B. (1961) *The Dynamics of Culture Change*, Westport, CT: Greenwood Press.

Mand, K. (2002) 'Place, gender and power in transnational Sikh marriages', 'Transnational households and rituals: an overview', *Global networks: a journal of transnational affairs*, July, 2, 3: 233–48.

Mand, K. (2006) *South Asian Families and Social Capital: Rituals of Care and Provision*, Families & Social Capital ESRC Research Group Working Paper Series, London: South Bank University.

Martiniello, M. and Lafleur, J. M. (2008) 'Towards a Transatlantic Dialogue in the Study of Immigrant Political Transnationalism', *Ethnic and Racial Studies*, 31, 4: 645–63.

Mason, J. (1999) 'Living Away from Relatives: Kinship and Geographical Reasoning', in S. McRae (ed.), *Changing Britain: Families and Households in the 1990s*, Oxford: Oxford University Press, 156–75.

Maynard, M. and Purvis, J. (eds) (1994) *Researching women's lives from a feminist perspective,* London: Taylor & Francis.

Messina, A. M. (2007) *The Logics and Politics of Post WWII Migration to Western Europe*, Cambridge: Cambridge University Press.

Medaglia, A. (2001) *Patriarchal Structures and Ethnicity in the Italian Community in Britain*, Aldershot: Ashgate.

Milbrath, L. W. (1965) *Political Participation*, Chicago: Rand McNally.

Miles, R. and Phizacklea, A. (1984) *White Man's Country: Racism in British Politics*, London: Pluto Press.

Millennium Development Report (2004) *Millennium Development Goals: Jamaica April 2004*, Kingston: The Planning Institute of Jamaica.

Mills, C. W. (1970) *The Sociological Imagination*, Harmondsworth: Penguin.

Modood, T. (2004) 'Capitals, Ethnic Identity and Educational Qualifications', *Cultural Trends*, 13, 2: 87–105.

Modood, T. (2007) *Multiculturalism*, Cambridge: Polity Press.

Modood, T., Berthoud, R., Lakey, J., Nazroo, J., Smith, P., Virdee, S. and Beishon, S. (eds) (1997) *Ethnic Minorities in Britain*, London: Policy Studies Institute.

Molyneaux, M. (2001) 'Social Capital: A Post Transition Concept?: questions of context and gender from Latin American perspectives', in V. Morrow (ed.), *An Appropriate Capitalisation?: questioning social capital*, Research in Progress Series, Issue 1, Special Issue, Gender Institute, London School of Economics.

Morokvasic, M. (1983) 'Women and Migration: beyond the reductionist outlook', in A. Phizacklea (ed.) *One Way Ticket: migration and female labour*, London: Routledge and Kegan Paul, 13–31.

Morokvasic, M. (1984) 'Birds of a passage are also women', *International Migration Review*, 18, 4: 886–907.

Morrow, V. (1999) 'Conceptualising Social Capital in Relation to the Well-Being of Children and Young People: A Critical Review, *Sociological Review*, 47, 4: 744–65.

Myrdal, G. (1944) *An American Dilemma: The Negro Problem and Modern Democracy*, New York: Harper and Row.

Myrdal, G. (1970) *Objectivity in Social Research*, London: Duckworth.

Nathan, D. (2007) 'Mauritian health workers returning from Britain', unpublished PhD thesis, London: South Bank University.

Nettleford, R. (2003) *Caribbean Cultural Identity: The Case of Jamaica, an Essay in Cultural Dynamics*, Jamaica: Ian Randle Publishers.

Nicholls, D. (1974) *Three Varieties of Pluralism*, London: Macmillan.

Ni Laoire, C. (2007) 'The "Green Green Grass of Home"? Return Migration to Rural Ireland', *Journal of Rural Studies*, 23, 3: 332–44.

Oakley, A. (1972) *Sex, Gender and Society*, London: Temple Smith.

Orr, M. (1999) *Black Social Capital: The Politics of School Reform in Baltimore, 1986–1998*, Kansas: University of Kansas Press.

Ostergaard-Nielsen, E. (2003) *Transnational Politics: Turks and Kurds in Germany*, London: Routledge.

Ouseley, H. (2001) *Community Pride, Not Prejudice: Making Diversity Work in Bradford*, Bradford: Bradford Vision.

Owen, D. (1994) 'Size, Structure and Growth of the Ethnic Minority Populations', in D Coleman and J Salt (eds), *Ethnicity in the 1991 Census: Demographic Characteristics of the Ethnic Minority Populations*, London: HMSO, 80–123.

Owen, D. (2001) 'A profile of Caribbean households and families in Great Britain', in H. Goulbourne and M. Chamberlain (eds) *Caribbean families in Britain and the trans-Atlantic world*, London: Macmillan, 64–95.

Owen, D. (2006) 'Demographic Profiles and Social Cohesion of Minority Ethnic Communities in England and Wales', *Community, Work and Family*, 9, 3: 251–72.

Pahl, R. (2000) *On Friendship*, Cambridge: Polity Press.

Pahl, R. and Pevalin, D. (2005) 'Between Family and Friends: A Longitudinal Study of Friendship Choice', *British Journal of Sociology*, 56, 3: 433–50.

Pahl, R., Pevalin, D. and Spencer, E. (2006) 'Friendships Over the Lifecourse', paper presented at British Sociological Association Annual Conference, International Centre, Harrogate, 22 April.

Palmer, R. (1977) 'The Italians: Patterns of Migration in London', in J. L. Watson (ed.), *Between Two Cultures. Migrants and Minorities in Britain*, Oxford: Basil Blackwell.

Panagakos, A. N. (2004) 'Recycled Odyssey: Creating Transnational Families in the Greek Diaspora', *Global Networks*, 4, 3: 299–311.

Parekh, B. (2000) *The Future of Multicultural Britain*, London: Runnymede Trust.

Park, R. E. (1950) *Race and Culture*, New York: The Free Press.

Parreñas, R. S. (2001) *Servants of Globalization: Women, Migration, and Domestic Work*, Stanford: Stanford University Press.

Parreñas, R. S. (2005) Children of Global Migration: Transnational Families and Gendered Woes, Stanford: Stanford University Press.

Patterson, S (1965) Dark Strangers: A Study of West Indians in London, Harmondsworth: Penguin.

Peach, C. (1968) *West Indian Migrants in Britain*, London: Oxford University Press.

Peach, C. (1991) 'The Caribbean in Europe: Contrasting Patterns of Migration and Settlement in Britain, France and the Netherlands', Coventry: Centre for Research in Ethnic Relations, University of Warwick, Research Paper 15.

Phillips, M. and Phillips, T. (1998) *Windrush: The Irresistible Rise of Multi-Cultural Britain*, New York: Harper Collins.

Phizacklea, A. (ed.) (1983) *One Way Ticket: migration and female labour*, London: Routledge and Kegan Paul.

Pilkington, E. (1988) *Beyond the Mother Country: West Indians and the Notting Hill White Riots*, London: I.B. Tauris.

Platt, L., Simpson, L. and Akinwale, B. (2005) 'Stability and Change in Ethnic Groups in England and Wales', *Population Trends*, 121: 35–46.

Plaza, D. (2000) 'In Pursuit of the Mobility Dream: Second-Generation British-Caribbeans Returning to Jamaica and Barbados', *Journal of Eastern Caribbean Studies*, 27, 4: 135–60.

Plaza, D. (2000) 'Transnational Grannies: The Changing Family Responsibilities of Elderly African Caribbean-Born Women Resident in Britain', *Social Indicators Research*, 51: 75–105

Plummer, K. (1993) 'Intimate Citizenship and the Culture of Sexual Story Telling', in

J. Weeks, J. Holland and M. Waites (eds), *Sexualities and Society: A Reader*, Oxford: Polity.

Plummer, K. (2003) *Intimate Citizenship: private decisions and public dialogues*, Montreal: McGill-Queen's University Press.

Portes, A. (1998) 'Social Capital: its Origin and Applications in Modern Sociology', *Annual Review of Sociology*, 24: 1–24.

Portes, A. (2001) 'Introduction: the Debates and Significance of Immigrant Transnationalism', *Global Networks*, 1, 3: 181–94.

Portes, A. and Zhou, M. (1993) 'The New Second Generation: Segmented Assimilation and its Variants Among Post-1965 Immigrant Youth', *Annals of the American Academy of Political Science*, 5, 30: 74–98.

Portes, A. and Zhou, M. (2001) 'The New Second Generation: Segmented Assimilation and its Variants', in H. Goulbourne (ed.) *Race and Ethnicity: critical concepts in sociology*, 4: 314–36.

Portes, A., Guranizo, L. and Landolt, P. (1999) 'The Study of Transnationalism: Pitfalls and Promise of an Emergent Research Field', Ethnic and Racial Studies, 22, 2: 217–37.

Portes, A., Escobar, C. and Arana, R. (2008) 'Bridging the Gap: Transnational and Ethnic Organizations in the Political Incorporation of Immigrants in the United States', *Ethnic and Racial Studies*, 31, 6: 1056–90.

Potter, R. B. (2005) ' "Young, Gifted and Back": Second-Generation Transnational Return Migrants to the Caribbean', *Progress in Development Studies*, 5, 3: 213–36.

Potter, R. B. and Phillips, J. (2006) 'Both Black and Symbolically White: The "Bajan-Brit" Return Migrant as a Post-Colonial Hybrid', *Ethnic and Racial Studies*, 29, 5: 901–27.

Potter, R. B., Conway, D. and Phillips, J. (eds) (2005) *The Experience of Return Migration: Caribbean Perspectives*, Aldershot: Ashgate.

Putnam, R. (1994) 'Tuning In, Tuning Out: the strange disappearance of social capital in America'. Available at: http://www.apsanet.org/imgtest/PSDec95Putnam.pdf (accessed 1 June, 2006).

Putnam, R. (2000) *Bowling Alone – The Collapse and Revival of American Community*, New York: Simon and Schuster.

Putnam, R. (2007) 'E Pluribus Unum: Diversity and Community in the Twenty-first Century. The 2006 Johan Skytte Prize Lecture', *Scandinavian Political Studies*, 30, 2: 137–74.

Rattansi, A. (2005) 'The Uses of Racialization: The Time-Spaces and Subject-Objects of the Raced Body', in K. Murji and J. Solomos (eds), *Racialization: Studies in Theory and Practice*, Oxford: Oxford University Press.

Reay, D. and Mirza, H. (1997) 'Uncovering Genealogies at the Margins: Black Supplementary Schools', *British Journal of Sociology of Education*, 18, 4: 477–99.

Rex, J. and Tomlinson, S. (1979) *Colonial Immigrants in a British City: A Class Analysis*, London: Routledge and Kegan Paul.

Reynolds, T (1997) '(Mis)Representing the Black (Super)Woman', in H. Mirza (ed.), *Black British Feminism: A Reader*, London: Routledge.

Reynolds, T. (2001) 'Black Mothering, Paid Work and Identity', *Ethnic and Racial Studies*, 24, 6: 1046–64.

Reynolds, T. (2003) 'Black to the Community: Black Community Parenting in the UK', *Community, Work and Family*, 6, 1: 29–41.

Reynolds, T. (2004) *Families, Social Capital and Caribbean Young People's Diasporic Identities*, Families & Social Capital ESRC Research Group, Working Paper No. 11, London: South Bank University.

Reynolds, T. (2005) *Caribbean Mothers: Identity and Experience in the UK*, London: Tufnell Press.

Reynolds, T. (2006a) 'Caribbean Young People, Family Relationships and Social Capital', *Ethnic and Racial Studies*, 29, 6: 1087–103.

Reynolds, T. (2006b) 'Bonding Social capital within the Caribbean Family and Community', *Community, Work and Family* 9, 3: 273–90.

Reynolds, T. (2007) 'Friendship Networks, Social Capital and Ethnic Identity: Researching the Perspectives of Caribbean Young People in Britain', *Journal of Youth Studies*, 10, 4: 383–98.

Reynolds, T. (2008) *Ties that Bind: Families, Social Capital and Caribbean Second-Generation Return Migration*, Brighton: University of Sussex, Sussex Centre for Migration Research Working Paper No. 46.

Reynolds, T. (forthcoming 2009) 'Exploring the Absent/Present Dilemma: Black Fathers, Family Relationships and Social Capital in Britain', *Annals of the American Academy of Political and Social Science.*

Reynolds, T. and Zontini, E. (2006) 'A Comparative Study of Care Provision Across Caribbean and Italian Transnational Families', Working Paper Series, Families and Social Capital ESRC Research Group, London: South Bank University.

Reynolds, T. and Miah, N. (2007) *Black Asian and Minority Ethnic Employment Skills*, London: Borough of Lambeth.

Rich, P. B. (1990) *Race and Empire in British Politics*, Cambridge: Cambridge University Press.

Robins, K. and Aksoy, A. (2001) 'From Spaces of Identity to Metnal Spaces: Lessons from the Turkish Cypriot Cultural Experience in Britain', *Journal of Ethnic and Migration Studies*, 27, 4: 685–711.

Rodriguez, R. M. (2008) '(Dis)unity and Diversity in Post–9/11 America', *Sociological Forum*, 23, 2: 379–89.

Roopnarine, J. and Brown, J. (eds) (1997) *Caribbean Families: Diversity Among Ethnic Groups*, London: JAI Press.

Roopnarine, J. and Gielen, U. (2005) *Families in Global Perspective*, Boston: Pearson Educational.

Runnymede Trust (2004) *Civic Renewal and Social Capital*, London: Runnymede Trust.

Ruston, D. (2001) *Social Capital: Matrix of Surveys*, London: Office of National Statistics.

Russel-Browne, P., Norville, B. and Griffith, C. (1997) 'Childshifting: a survival strategy for teenage mothers', in J. Roopnarine and J. Brown (eds) *Caribbean families: diversity amongst groups*, Norwood, New Jersey: Ablex Publishing.

Scarman, L. (1981) *The Brixton Disorders 10–12 April 1981. Report of an Inquiry by the Rt. Hon. The Lord Scarman OBE*, London: HMSO.

Scarman, L. (1985) 'Brixton and After', in J. Roach and J. Thomaneak (eds), *Police and Public Order in Europe*, London: Croom Helm, 7–14.

Schattschneider, E. E. (1967) *The Semi-sovereign People: a realist view of democracy in America*, 2nd ed, New York: Holt, Rhinhart and Winston.

Schuster, L. (2003) *The Use and Abuse of Political Asylum in Britain and Germany*, London: Frank Cass.

Schuster, L. and Solomos, J. (2004) 'Race, Immigration and Asylum: New Labour's Agenda and its Consequences', *Ethnicities*, 4, 2: 267–300.

Sciama, L. (2003) *A Venetian Island: Environment, History and Change in Burano*, Oxford: Berghahn Books.

Senior, O. (1991) *Working Miracles: Women's Lives in the English Speaking Caribbean*, London: James Currey Publishing.

Sevenhuijsen, S. (2000) 'Caring in the Third Way: The Reflection between Obligation, Responsibility and Care in the Third Way Discourse', *Critical Social Policy*, 20, 1: 5–37.

Sewell, T. (1997) *Black Masculinities and Schooling: How Black Boys Survive Modern Schooling*, London: Trentham Books.

Shaha, B. (2007) 'Being Young, Female and Laotian: Ethnicity as Social Capital at the Intersection of Gender, Generation, "Race" and Age', *Ethnic and Racial Studies*, 30, 1: 28–50.

Silva, E. B. and Smart, C. (eds) (1999) *The New Family?*, London: Sage.

Sivanandan, A. (1982) *A Different Hunger: Writings on Black Resistance*, London: Pluto Press.

Sivanandan, A. (1990) *Communities of Resistance: Writings on Black Struggles for Socialism*, London: Verso.

Skeggs, B. (1997) *Formations of Class and Gender*, London: Sage.

Smart, C. (2007) *Personal Life*, Cambridge: Polity Press.

Smart, C. and Shipman, B. (2004) 'Visions in Monochrome: Families, Marriage and the Individualization Thesis', *British Journal of Sociology*, 55, 4: 491–509.

Smith, A. M. (1994) *New Right Discourse on Race and Sexuality: 1968–1990*, Cambridge: Cambridge University Press.

Smith, M. G. (1962a) *The Plural Society in the British West Indies*, Los Angeles: University of California Press.

Smith, M. G. (1962b) *West Indian Family Structure*, Seattle and London: University of Washington Press.

Smith, R. T. (1953) *The Matrifocal Family*, London: Routledge and Kegan Paul.

Smith, R. T. (1956) *The Negro Family in British Guiana: family structure and social status in the villages*, London: Routledge and Kegan Paul.

Smith, R. T. (2001) 'Caribbean Families: questions for research and implications for policy', in H. Goulbourne and M. Chamberlain (eds) *Caribbean families in Britain and the trans-Atlantic world*, London: Macmillan, 48–62.

Smith, R. T. (1996) *The Matrifocal Family: Power, Politics and Pluralism*, rev. edn, London: Routledge.

Solomos, J. (1991) *Black Youth, Racism and the State: The Politics of Ideology and Policy*, Cambridge: Cambridge University Press.

Solomos, J. (2003) *Race and Racism in Britain*, 3rd edn, Basingstoke: Palgrave Macmillan.

Solomos, J. and Back, L. (1996) *Racism and Society*, London: St Martin's Press.

Solomos, J. and Bulmer, M. (eds) (1999) *Racism*, Oxford: Oxford University Press.

Song, M. and Edwards, R. (1997) 'Comment: Raising Questions about Perspectives on Black Lone Motherhood', *Journal of Social Policy*, 26, 2: 23–44.

Stasiulis, D. and Ross, D. (2006) 'Security, Flexible Sovereignty, and the Perils of Multiple Citizenship', *Citizenship Studies*, 10, 3: 329–48.

Strategy Unit (2003) *Ethnic Minorities in the Labour Market*, London: Strategy Unit.

Sutton, C. (2004) 'Celebrating Ourselves: The Family Rituals of African-Caribbean Transnational Families', *Global Networks*, 4, 3: 243–57.

Swan, Lord Michael (1985) Education for All: Report of the Committee of Inquiry into the Education of Children from Minority Ethnic Groups, Cmnd 9453, London: HMSO.

Swedberg, R. (2003) 'The Changing Picture of Max Weber's Sociology', *Annual Review of Sociology*, 29, 1: 283–306.

Thomas-Hope, E. (ed.) (2009) *Freedom and Constraint in Caribbean Migration and Diaspora*, Kingston: Ian Randle Publishers.

Thompson, P. (1978) *The voice of the past: oral history*, Oxford: Oxford University Press.

Thorne, B. and Yalom, M. (eds) (1992) *Rethinking the Family: Some Feminist Questions*, Boston: Northern University Press.

Tonnies, F. (1955) *Community and Association* (trans. C. P. Loomis), London: Routledge and Kegan Paul.

Trotz, D. A. (2006) 'Rethinking Caribbean Transnational Connections: Conceptual Itineraries', *Global Networks*, 6, 1: 41–59.

Tubito, M. and King, R. (1996) 'Italians in Peterborough: between integration and return', *Research Paper 27*, Brighton: University of Sussex.

Vansina, J. (1965) *Oral tradition: a study in historical methodology*, Harmondsworth: Penguin.

Vasta, E. (1993) 'Cultural and social change: Italo-Australian women and the second generation', *Altreitalie*, 9: 69–83.

Vertovec, S. (2007) 'Super-Diversity and its Implications', *Ethnic and Racial Studies*, 30, 6: 1024–54.

Vickerman, M. (1999) *Crosscurrents: West Indian Immigrants and Race*, Oxford: Oxford University Press.

Ward, R. and Jenkins, R. (eds) (1984) *Ethnic Communities in Business: Strategies for Economic Survival*, Cambridge: Cambridge University Press.

Waters, M. (1999) Black Identities: West Indian Immigrants, Dreams and Realities, Cambridge, MA: Harvard University Press.

Weber, M. (1995) *Max Weber: selections in translation*, W. G. Runciman (ed.), E. Matthews (tr.), Cambridge: Cambridge University Press.

Weeks, J. (2007) *The World We Have Won*, London: Routledge.

Weller, S. and Bruegel, I. (2006) *Locality, School and Social Capital: Findings Report*, Families & Social Capital ESRC Research Group, London: South Bank University.

Werbner, P. (2002) *Imagined Diasporas Among Manchester Muslims: The Public Performance of Pakistani Transnational Identity Politics*, Oxford: James Currey.

Werbner, P. (2004) 'Theorising Complex Diasporas: Purity and Hybridity in the South Asian Public Sphere in Britain', *Journal of Ethnic and Migration Studies*, 30, 5: 895–911.

Wessendorf, S. (2007) '"Roots Migrants": Transnationalism and "Return" Among Second-Generation Italians in Switzerland', *Journal of Ethnic and Migration Studies*, 33, 7: 1083–102.

Western, J. (1992) *A Passage to England: Barbadian Londoners Speak of Home*, London: UCL Press.

Wetherell, M., Lafleche, M. and Berkeley, R. (eds) (2007) *Identity, Ethnic Diversity and Community Cohesion*, London: Sage.

Williams, F. (2005) *Rethinking Families*, London: Calouste Gulbenkian Foundation.

Wolf, D. (2004) 'Valuing Informal Elder Care', in N. Folbre and M. Bittman (eds), *Family Time: the social organization of care*, London: Routledge.

Woolcock, M (1998) 'Some Conceptual and Economic Developments: Towards a Theoretical Synthesis and Policy Framework', *Theory and Society*, 27, 2: 151–208.

Yates, N. (2009) *Migrant Care Workers: Nurses, Nuns and Nannies*, London: Palgrave Macmillan.

Zhou, M. (1997) 'Segmented Assimilation: Issues, Controversies, and Recent Research on the New Second Generation', *International Migration Review*, 31, 4: 179–91.

Zontini, E. (2004a) 'Immigrant Women in Barcelona: Coping with the Consequences of Transnational Lives', *Journal of Ethnic and Migration Studies*, 30, 6: 1113–44.

Zontini, E. (2004b) *Italian Families and Social Capital: Rituals and the Provision of Care in British-Italian Transnational Families*, Families & Social Capital ESRC Research Group, Working Paper Series, No. 6, London: South Bank University.

Zontini, E. (2006) 'Italian Families and Social Capital: Care Provision in a Transnational World', *Community, Work and Family*, 9, 3: 325–45.

Zontini, E. (2008) 'Dreaming of "Home" and "Belonging" in Transnational Families: Generational Views on "Return"', Paper presented at the 10th EASA Biennial Conference, Ljubljana, 26–30 August.

Zontini, E. (2009) *Transnational Families, Migration and Gender: Moroccan and Filipino Women in Bologna and Barcelona*, Oxford: Berghahn Books.

Index

alienation 135–7, 143–4, 149, 151
altruism, prescribed 96
anti-immigration ideologies 51
anti-racism 57
Arneil, Barbara 29
asylum seekers 51, 54, 56, 58, 60
autonomy 17, 23, 82
Aylesbury 40, 91, 108

babysitting 89–90, 134, 142, 163
Barbados, interviews in 40
Bedford 19–20, 40, 70–1, 91, 105, 108, 114, 143
biases 38–9, 44
Bourdieu, Pierre 28–9, 136

Calabrians 19
capital: different forms of 31; social *see* social capital
Caribbean communities: divisions between 155–8, 164; ethnic identity of 100–1, 145–50; and ethnic mixing 164–7; and ethnic mixing 164–7; and food 109; and football 117–18; gender roles in 152–3, 159–60; holidays in 102–4; integration of 110–11; interview subjects 40; neighbourhoods 66–8; parenting in 79, 107, 161–2, 172; and political engagement 32; and research 44; return migration 69–70, 84–5, 87–8, 120–1, 123–5, 131–2; role of family in 82; settlement patterns of 65–6; visits to homeland 86, 103
caring: about 83–4; boundaries and obligations 94–7; dependency model of 82; for 87, 92–3, 112; and friendship networks 91–2; international 179–80; types of 13, 81, 83
childcare 65, 87–8, 92, 153
children: of Caribbean migrants 57, 66, 68–9, 76–8, 86–8, 100–1, 103, 106–7, 111, 116, 118, 125, 132–3, 146–51, 160; of Caribbean migrants 57, 66, 68–9, 76–8, 86–8, 100–1, 103, 106–7, 111, 116, 118, 125, 132–3, 146–51, 160; of Italian migrants 71–2, 74–5,

86, 89, 112, 126, 133–4; of Italian migrants 71–2, 74–5, 86, 89, 112, 126, 133–4; of mixed families 173; relationship with parents 19, 82, 84, 87, 95–6; and religion 107; and return migration 124–5
Christmas 84, 102–5, 173
citizenship 34, 49–50, 99, 113
communities: and families 23; purpose of 24
community, sense of 28–9
conflict: contagious 42; intergenerational 19
cultural differences 25, 82, 132, 135, 162, 167, 171, 173
cultural remittances 84, 94
culture contact 25, 33
culture shock 129, 133

diasporas 4–5, 99–100, 119, 125, 128
dis-trust 29
divorce 89, 134, 137–8, 171
Durkheim, Émile 24, 31, 38

Easter 84, 102, 104–5, 173
education: discrimination in 53; and ethnic diversity 68–9
elderly people: care of 142–3; in Caribbean community 90, 95–6; in Italian communities 73, 91, 96, 108
emotional blackmail 139–40
employment: of Caribbean people 80, 158–9; discrimination in 53, 59; and immigration policy 56
English accent 114, 127, 131–2, 152
ESRC (Economic and Social Research Council) 15n1, 179
ethnic communities: in America 32–3; and public policy 57–9; value systems of 32
ethnic identity: in America 34, 68; and community organizations 24, 108; formation of 78, 100, 108, 119, 144–5; and higher education 80; and media images 116; multiple 172–4; and racism 27; and religion 105–6; and social cohesiveness 67; and

success 148; understanding of 113
ethnicity: definition of 25; and friendship 73,
    75–7, 79, 113–14; of interviewer 44–5; and
    race 26; regional 45; as social capital 13–14,
    32, 35; vagueness of concept 30

families: Caribbean 21–3, 84, 96, 124, 136,
    138, 141, 144–5, 165, 179; dispersal of 10,
    82; ethical questions for researchers 46; and
    identity 101; Italian 17–18, 109, 179; mixed
    9, 155, 165, 172–3, 175; negotiations in 96;
    nuclear 19, 23; purpose of 24; reciprocal
    relationships in 82, 178; rituals of 47,
    101–2; role of women in 140–1; and social
    system 17; tensions and conflicts in 136–44,
    146–9, 178–9
family networks 20, 82, 84, 90, 100–1, 128, 153
family values 141
fathers: in Caribbean families 21–2; in Italian
    families 19
feminism 21, 37, 81, 83, 136, 144
food 71, 76, 85, 88, 93, 95, 109–10, 117, 152,
    171
friendship 14, 22, 46, 65, 73–80, 91–2, 113,
    132, 147, 151; networks 46, 69, 73, 77, 80,
    91, 113, 130, 153, 178, 181
fronticring 7–8

gatekeepers 43–4, 47
gay and lesbian people 17, 29, 41, 74, 161
gemeinschaft and *gesellschaft* 23–4
gender 3, 6, 12, 23, 36, 83, 97, 115, 129, 149,
    157, 178, 180
generation/s: care between 87, 142, 178;
    change between 80, 178; cohesion between
    18, 20; conflict between 19, 137; crossing
    of boundaries 3; differences between 84,
    93, 116, 124; experience of 37; and family
    networks 101; and identity 6, 12, 36,
    83, 180; learning between 88, 109; links
    between 65–6, 82, 85, 94, 103, 121, 135,
    142–3; migrant 69, 71, 106, 117, 127; norms
    of 141; and poverty 68; returnee 127; risks
    to 23; second and third 14, 19–20, 57, 73,
    115; and social mobility 111
gift-giving 84–5
globalization 3–5, 9, 13, 16, 29, 60, 99, 120
grandparents 22, 65, 84, 87–90, 110, 126, 142,
    145, 166, 170, 173
guilt 87, 91, 95, 137, 142–3, 154, 174
Guyana, interviews in 40

homophobia 160–2
housing, discrimination in 53
hybridization 131

identity: black 146, 148, 150, 154; blurring
    178; children's formation of 75, 77, 79;
collective 10, 24, 100, 145, 150; cultural 11,
    79, 85, 100–1, 111, 115, 136–7, 144, 146;
    ethnic *see* ethnic identities; evolution of 25;
    Italian 101, 105, 109, 114; local 66; multiple
    12, 60, 100, 113, 118, 180; national 26,
    37, 99, 103, 116–18; racial 3, 13, 26–7, 36,
    79–80, 111, 165; supranational 114–15; and
    transnational experience 6, 83, 99–100
immigrant communities 4, 14, 20, 33
individualism 18, 23, 81–2
Indo-Caribbeans 165–6
integration 11, 18, 32–3, 53, 60, 65, 110–11,
    118, 127, 153
Internet 9, 84–5, 88, 94
interviews, as research tools 41
Irish community 32, 52, 120
Islam 75, 136, 173
Italian communities: cultural values of 19–20;
    divisions between 162–3; and ethnic mixing
    167–71; and family structure 18; and food
    109–10; and football 117–18; gender roles
    in 163; integration of 111–13; national and
    regional identity of 45; return migration
    121–4, 126–30; role of family in 82;
    settlement patterns of 70–2; social networks
    of 43; visits to homeland 85–7, 90

Jamaica, interviews in 40
Jewish community 32, 51

kin-keeping 84–5, 92, 94
kinship: care 81; groups 3, 17, 23–4, 32–3, 60,
    84, 155, 166, 178; morality 83, 95; networks
    9, 13–14, 16–17, 22–4, 30, 40, 83, 101, 113,
    155–6; responsibilities 96
knife-grinders 70, 126–8

language 24–6, 44, 166–7, 171, 173
learning, inter-generational 88
letters 42, 83, 93, 121, 144, 179
London, interviews in 40
Lummis, Trevor 41

marginalization 83, 111–12
marriage: in Caribbean communities 21–2; in
    Italian communities 112, 128, 163–4; mixed
    166–8, 171, 173–5
Marx, Karl 24, 30–1
Mauritius 120
media 52, 56, 60, 116, 149
migration: current focus on 60; and family
    relationships 81; history of 50–5; Italian 18,
    70; to North America 124; racialization of
    55–7; research on 49–50
modernity 9, 13, 22
multiculturalism 14, 16, 34, 37, 50, 56, 59, 61,
    116, 180
Myrdal, Gunnar 38–9, 47, 179

nation, as imagined community 5–6, 23
nation-states 3–5, 8–13, 16, 36–7, 99
negotiations 7–8, 42–3, 96–7, 136, 164, 178
Notting Hill 52, 56, 113
Nottingham 40, 52, 56, 70, 104, 145, 175

objectivity 37–9
old age 6
oral history method 41–2

Pakistani community 4, 84, 114, 121
parenting 21, 140–1, 161
Peterborough 40, 70, 75, 91, 94, 105, 108, 143
Plummer, Ken 41
poverty 58, 68, 92, 130, 147, 158
Putnam, Robert 28–9, 34

race: and ethnicity 26; and migration 53; riots
    52, 56
race relations 50–1, 58–9
Race Relations Act 53–4, 58–9
racial discrimination 51, 53, 57, 59, 67, 77,
    86, 159
racism, institutionalized 57–9, 107
reciprocity 13, 19, 34, 43, 46, 82, 103
refugees 51–2, 54, 60
relationships: intimate 17, 23–4, 162, 164, 181;
    social 19, 23, 124–5, 128
relativizing 7
religion 25–6, 45, 109, 166, 171, 174; and
    Caribbean community 104, 106–8, 158; and
    Italian community 43, 45, 75, 105–6, 108;
    and Italian community 43, 45, 75, 105–6,
    108
remittances 4, 93–4, 130
Rendena valley 72, 125–6
research process 42, 44, 46–7
research questions 35–6, 39
retirement 120, 123
Ribera 71, 106, 121–3, 130–1, 133–4

sacrifice 19, 95, 122, 130, 135n1, 142
sacrifici see sacrifice
school: and Caribbean children 21–2, 77–8,
    92, 146; and Italian children 74, 143–4;
    racial inequalities in 68; supplementary
    106–7, 148
Second World War 52, 65, 70, 162
self-censorship 116
sexual morality 157
sexuality 3, 6, 150–1, 161
siblings 82, 84–5, 87, 92–3, 126, 139, 159, 166
Sicily 40, 105, 121–4, 129–30, 134, 142, 164
social action 13, 26–8, 32, 36, 38–9, 179
social capital: bonding 31–2, 45, 67; bridging
    45, 67; community 14; in daily life 47–8n1;
    and ethnic identity 113; and families 137,

143; identification of 30; key issue in
    social science 16; literature on 27–31; and
    remittances 94; and research 44, 47; and
    return migration 128, 131–2; theory of
    12–14; types of 31; vagueness of concept
    30–1
social change 14, 41, 150, 155
social class: and ethnicity 147–50, 157, 162;
    and experience of transnationalism 6; and
    identity choices 115; and international travel
    91; mobility in 92; and schooling 77–9; and
    social capital 28; and women's clubs 108
social exclusion 34, 99–100, 110, 112
social fields 12, 120, 178
social mobility, upward 22, 66–8, 71, 111,
    122–4, 147, 150, 158–9
social networks 34, 44–5, 65, 73, 78–9, 91, 99,
    107, 113
social remittance 94
socialization 24, 131
solidarity 18–20, 34–5, 37, 96, 108–9, 111–12,
    130–1, 143–4
South Asians 21, 24, 26, 165–6, 179
subjectivity 38–41, 99
Sylhetis 4

Thatcher, Margaret 54, 57
Thompson, Paul 41
transnational experiences 4–6, 9, 13, 164, 177,
    181
transnational families: boundaries of 9; and
    caring 81, 83–4; communication in 36;
    connections of 11; cross-boundaries of 12;
    networks 93, 100, 119; relationships in 123;
    research on 3–8
transnational individual 10
transnational networks 43, 59, 99, 125, 175,
    181
transnational practices 128
transnationalism 5–7, 10–11, 13, 83, 122; from
    above 10; imperial 5
Trentino 40, 43, 72, 124, 126–30, 163
trust: in Italian families 19; and social capital
    30; in transnational families 84

university 44, 68–9, 71, 78–80, 143–4, 146,
    168, 171

Weber, Max 24, 38–9, 47
women: in Caribbean communities 21, 135,
    138–40, 151–2, 157–60; and caring 92–5;
    and Christmas celebrations 105; clubs for
    108; in Italian communities 19–21, 46, 71,
    73, 89, 129, 131, 133–5, 138, 140–1, 143–4,
    163, 169; and media images 116; and
    religion 107
World Cup 116–18